marie claire

real
achievable beauty for real women
beauty

EMMA BANNISTER

QUADRILLE

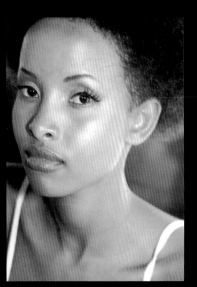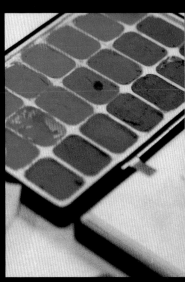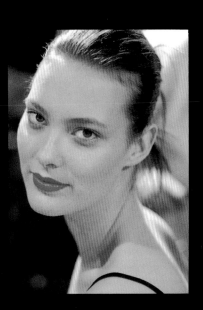

contents

introduction

Everyone is beautiful in their own way. Vitality, confidence and individuality are the bywords of modern beauty. While supermodel looks and the latest catwalk crazes can be inspirational, in **Real Beauty** we aim to show that it is great skin, healthy hair and make-up that reflects your personality that are the essence of real beauty.

Reassessing your features and routines is the first step to fulfilling your beauty potential. To help you, we asked five real women, representing a range of skin and hair types, to have their skin, hair and make-up problems analysed. Follow them through the book, as they undergo a series of makeovers, and in the process pick up practical advice, skills and guidance for use at home.

No book on beauty would be complete without addressing the issue of ageing and the way it affects women today. And although youth and beauty aren't one and the same thing, we now know so much about protecting our skin that a radiant youthful-looking complexion is something we can all aspire to.

Recent scientific advances mean that cosmetics have never been so easy to use. Nor have they ever been so plentiful. From glide-on foundations through translucent nail varnishes to anti-ageing night creams, the range is enormous and ever-growing. Marie Claire Real Beauty cuts through the mass of sometimes confusing information to show which products form the basis of a good skin- or haircare routine, which make-up formulations suit you best, and how they should be used. Ever wondered how make-up professionals achieve such perfect results? We give you the tools and expertise to enable you to create the image of your choice, saving you from time-consuming and costly mistakes and guaranteeing you a perfect finish.

Marie Claire Real Beauty is designed to give you the inspiration, knowledge and confidence to look your best. And remember, if you look good, you'll feel good too.

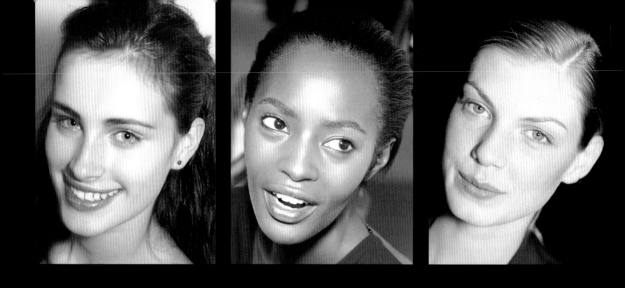

the
real you

YOUR beauty PERSONALITY

Your approach to beauty often mirrors your general attitude to life and, as such, reveals more about you than you realize. The quiz below is a light-hearted way of identifying your beauty 'personality', but working out which category you fall into may help you reassess your routine. Does it need updating, overhauling or simply paring down?

You are a beauty hoarder if

- you have more than ten shades of lipstick
- you keep more than two make-up bags permanently full
- you have kept a beauty sample from a magazine for longer than five months in the knowledge that you will use it at some point
- you have over 30 skincare and make-up products in your bathroom cabinet

You are a beauty minimalist if

- you use brown eyeliner pencil to outline your lips as well as your eyes
- petroleum jelly is your only source of lipstick, eyebrow gel, eyelash treatment and skin moisturiser
- you cleanse and tone your face with a face flannel and water, and nothing else
- you think a foundation is a Victorian undergarment
- you don't own a make-up bag because you don't have enough to put in it

You are living in the past if

- you apply your make-up just as you did ten years ago
- you have repurchased the same lip colour more than ten times
- your favourite lipstick shade has been discontinued
- you don't know that lip glosses now come in grown-up shades and not just cola-flavoured roll-ons

You are a beauty eclectic if

- you wear blue eyeshadow and red lipstick at the same time
- you wear just lip gloss one day and spend 30 minutes applying a perfect base the next
- you go shopping for cleanser and come home with nail polish and mascara instead
- you buy a lip colour because it looked good on the cover of a magazine
- you change your fragrance because someone sprays you with a new one in a department store

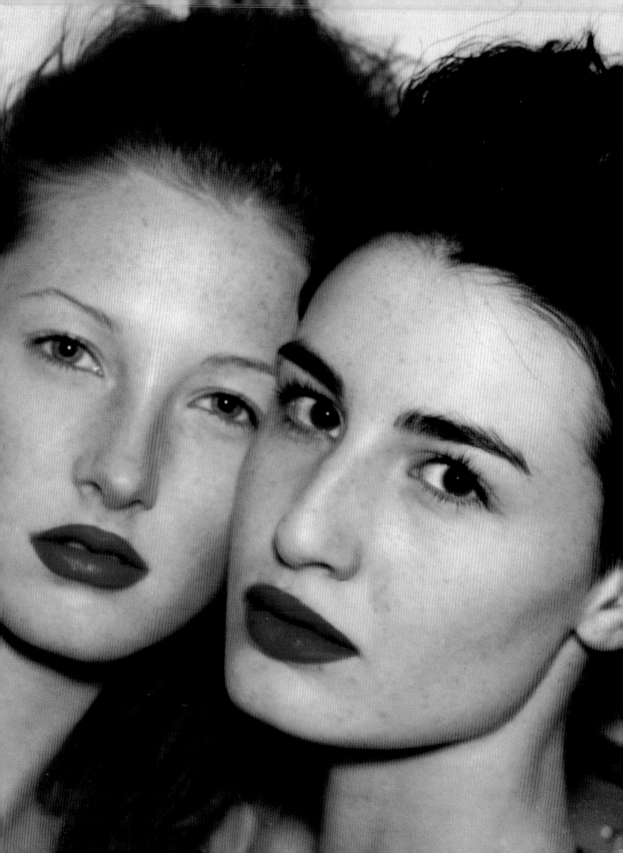

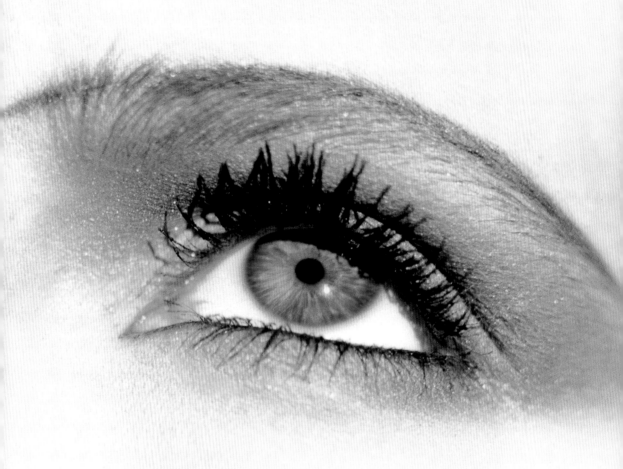

ANALYSE YOUR
face

Before embarking on a hair and make-up reassessment, take a good, long look at your face in the mirror. We catch our own reflections dozens of times every day but we rarely pause for thought and study our faces in depth. And yet an appreciation of their shape, structure and features will make it so much easier to emphasize strong points – large eyes, perhaps, or perfect bone structure – and to minimize the less flattering aspects, such as thin lips or a prominent chin. Your face shape, be it long and thin, square or round, can also be enhanced with a few subtle changes to your hair and make-up.

Symmetry is thought to be one of the keys to a beautiful face, so try to identify any imbalances in yours before you make any radical decisions. There are a number of ways of doing this. According to the ancient Greeks, the perfect face should divide horizontally into equal thirds: from the hairline to the eyebrows, from the brows to the base of the nose, and from there to the bottom of the chin. While we don't prize such classic, uniform proportions today, this approach still provides some useful guidelines for shading, blushing and highlighting.

Cosmetic surgeons have a different set of criteria – they tend to count a slightly domed forehead, a slim chin, a nose that is as long as the forehead is deep and eyes that are eye-width apart as the defining features of a beautiful face.

But perfection shouldn't really be your goal – individuality is one of the keys to real beauty and even the supermodels have their little flaws. What an awareness of your face and features can do is to show you how you can use simple make-up tricks to deflect attention from the features you hate while making the most of the ones you love, without going anywhere near a surgeon's knife.

For an objective view of yourself, get a friend to take a front-on polaroid photograph of you from two to three feet away. Don't laugh or pull a face; just keep your face as expressionless and relaxed as possible. A photograph such as this will draw your attention to uneven areas that you just don't notice when you look at yourself in the mirror.

Alternatively, white out your face with pale foundation. Then trace around your eyes and lips with a finely sharpened black kohl pencil to reveal your eye and lip shape. This will show you whether your features are balanced or if, for example, your top lip needs building with lip liner.

Eyebrows, the frame of a face, play an important role in facial symmetry. You can check their alignment by holding a straight, narrow object, such as an orange stick, against the edge of your nostril. The inner edge of the eyebrow should meet the top of the stick and, if you rotate it slightly towards the hairline, it should follow the outer edge of your eyebrows.

If you have an asymmetric haircut, brush your hair away from your face and tie it back before you study your features. If you have a side parting, try moving it from one side to the other – it may work better with your features. This is one of the best ways of finding out whether one side of your face is a little longer than the other.

Finding the right mirror

- Choose a mirror made from fairly thick glass – the reflection will be more accurate.
- Invest in a triple-view mirror so that you can get a really good look at yourself from all angles.
- Check your mirror is absolutely vertical when you examine your reflection, as a slanting perspective can distort it.

ANALYSE YOUR
skin

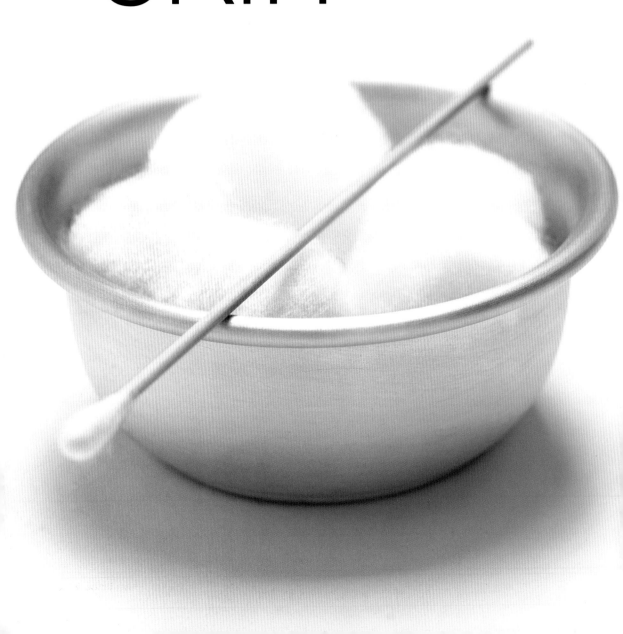

Skin is our largest functioning organ, and its condition reflects our lifestyle, skincare habits and general health. It tends to be categorized by its degree of oiliness. Oily skin usually goes hand in hand with open pores and will benefit from a gentle regime. Pores become more prominent after puberty and are linked to stress-related hormonal activity in the body. This is because stress triggers the production of androgen, the hormone that controls the size and secretion of the oil-producing glands.

Normal skin is the easiest to care for. It is usually plump and evenly coloured, but may have a slightly oily panel across the nose, chin and forehead, or T-zone. The presence of oily patches means this type of skin is often described as combination.

Dry skin is characterized by dry patches, but these may also be present in a dehydrated skin, which is quite different. Dry skin doesn't retain moisture well as it produces few protective oils, whereas dehydrated skin is a symptom of an overall drought in your system. Drinking plenty of water is advisable whatever your skin type, but it is particularly important if you have dehydrated skin. Signs of dehydration include ultra-fine criss-cross lines over areas such as the cheeks. Another indication is the presence of oily areas; truly dry skin will have no visible surface oil at all.

Sensitive skin tends to be fair and fragile, and should be treated with care. It is easily irritated and may have signs of surface redness and dry patches, where the skin has started to flake. Mature skin, on the other hand, is not a specific type but it does have some common characteristics. The most obvious are surface lines and wrinkles, but it can also be identified by a gradual decrease in firmness and spring, caused mainly by sun damage.

Blackheads, which are sometimes called comedones, occur when sebum produced in the skin dries and hardens before it reaches the surface, blocking the pores in the process. Dirt is then trapped in the oily plug, making it look black. The causes of blackheads include an oily skin in a drying environment, an unthorough cleansing routine and poor circulation, which can be boosted with massage and exercise. Try the new pore-cleansing strips, which are more gentle than metal extraction tools.

Spots and pimples are usually the result of bacteria penetrating the skin and causing infection. This produces the redness and inflammation we typically associate with spots and blemishes.

Acne is thought to be triggered by hormonal changes that occur during puberty and times of stress. When this happens, levels of androgen rise and the sebaceous glands go into overdrive. This results in the production of excessive amounts of oil, which ultimately leads to spots.

Blemish outbreaks in the chin and jaw area are usually attributed to stress and hormonal imbalances, whether they are caused by acne or not. If you suffer in this way, try changing your contraceptive pill (which affects your hormone levels), cutting down on caffeine-based drinks and junk foods, and indulge in a facial to boost lymphatic drainage.

Get to know your skin

- Touch is a great way of assessing your skin. Run slightly oily fingers over your entire face – your fingertips will pick up any rough, dry patches, as well as any bumps that are lurking below the surface.
- A magnifying mirror is a useful skincare tool as it will help you scrutinize your face at close quarters. Enlarged pores will be particularly obvious on the central panels of the cheeks, while any blackheads will be visible in the nose area. You may also spot broken capillaries over your cheekbones.
- Having your skin scanned by computer is a service that's offered free of charge by many beauty companies, which have the machines in selected department stores. A computer analysis will reveal the skin's fine surface lines, as well as the signs of sun damage, which will look like large, dark freckled areas.

ANALYSE YOUR
hair

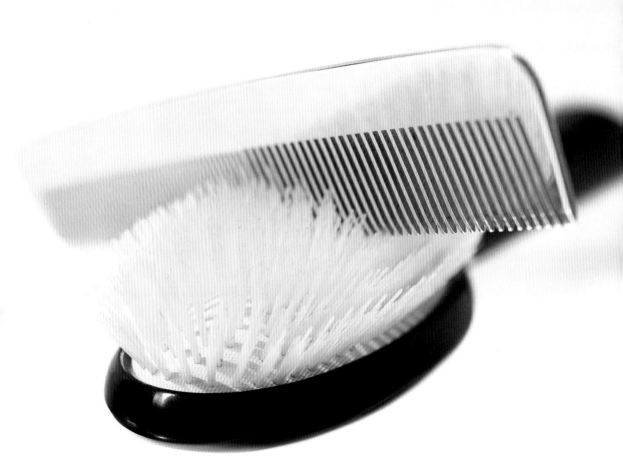

Analysing your hair to find out more about its condition, type and health isn't difficult and can certainly be done without technical gadgets. It's actually more about touch and observation than it is about science. And although many of the problems you discover can be remedied by changing either your products or your styling routine, you may also need to reconsider your diet and lifestyle if your hair is really dull and lifeless. Like skin, hair needs to be nourished and if you are run-down, the chances are that your hair is, too.

If you haven't identified your hair type correctly, you may also be using the wrong shampoos, conditioners and styling products, which means you probably aren't making the most of it. There are three basic types. Fine hair, which is usually troubled by static, shouldn't be confused with hair that's thinning or sparse. If your hair is fine, it isn't the quantity but the actual breadth of each strand that is the problem. So while you may have plenty of hair, the diameter of the hair shaft and its surrounding cuticles will be smaller than that of someone with normal hair. Thick hair, however, isn't a specific type – it simply refers to the number of hairs on your head and can be fine, oily or dry.

Oily hair, like oily skin, is the result of overactive sebaceous glands, but this time it is those in the scalp that are producing too much oil. Stress is a contributing factor, and the situation is often made worse by frequent washing, brushing and fiddling, all of which will further stimulate the oil-producing glands.

Dry hair is easy to identify. Run your fingers down through your hair, hold the ends and then run your fingers back up over its surface. If it feels rough, it is probably dry and in need of a nourishing treatment or oil. If you have coarse or frizzy hair, you'll probably find that it's also prone to dryness.

Once you have identified your hair type, focus on its condition. If, for example, your hair looks dull however frequently you wash it, you are probably overloading it with cleansing, conditioning and styling products. Give it a breather for a couple of weeks by using an ultra-mild shampoo and nothing else. Avoid styling mousses, gels and sprays as far as possible, as these will leave a residue on the surface of the hair, making the cuticles stand away from the hair shaft and the hair itself appear dull.

To assess the strength of your hair, take a strand between your fingertips and pull it taut. Strong, healthy hair is slightly elastic and should give a little under pressure. If it snaps easily it has probably been weakened by heat damage.

Cut down your use of hairdryers and heated appliances if you think your hair is fragile, or apply a heat-protective product first.

To identify split ends, stand against a bright light or window and study your hair. Any shorter strands standing out from the main body of your hair are likely to be broken ends. To check on the condition of long hair, grasp the ends and hold them against the roots. Any breakdown of condition and colour will be immediately obvious, indicating the need for either a new colour treatment or a good trim.

Flatter your face shape

- Your haircut, like your make-up, can enhance the shape of your face and, therefore, has an impact on your overall appearance. Oblong faces look great with jaw-length cuts. A blunt fringe is another way of breaking up a face that can look long and thin.
- Square faces will seem even more angular with blunt styles, so try a feathery cut instead, to soften any hard edges.
- If you have an oval face, most hair lengths and styles will suit you. Long, one-length hair is perhaps the only thing you should avoid, as it can create an unflattering triangular shape.

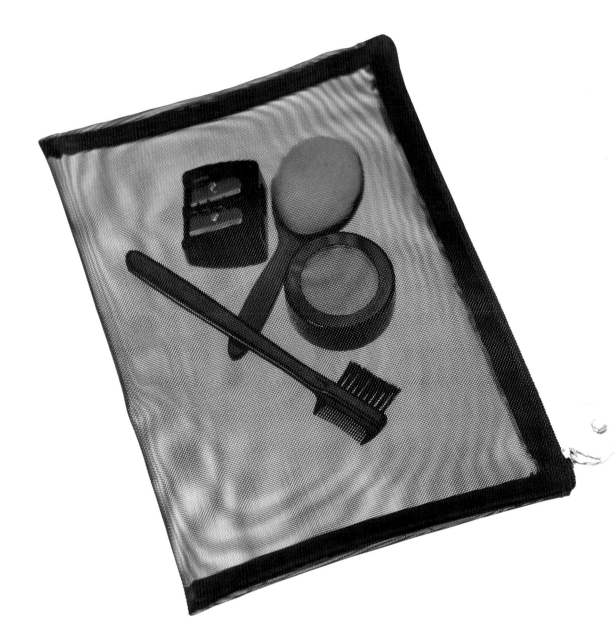

make-up bag

The average make-up bag is a good indicator of its owner's personality and frame of mind, as well as her make-up preferences. And, like most things, it will benefit from a thorough review every six months or so.

How many lip colours do you own? You probably don't need, or wear, more than two as most of us rely on one good shade for day and one for evening. Whittle out the rest or invest in a compact lip palette and decant your six favourite shades into it.

Reassess your impulse buys. Ask yourself honestly when you last wore each item, then discard any you haven't touched for months – you can't have been that impressed with them. And only keep the products that are right for the time of year in your make-up bag. Colours and textures that looked wonderful in the summer are probably completely wrong for the grey winter light; you may even find that you go off them altogether from one year to the next.

No one wants to carry around more than they need, so make the most of the wide range of dual-purpose products that are now available – they really earn their keep. Compact powder foundations, for example, are great for touching up bases and won't cause landslides of loose powder in your bag. Large, chunky crayon sticks, made by many beauty houses, can be used to add colour to lips, cheeks and eyes, while lip balm is a great all-rounder. Use it to highlight cheek- and browbones, to groom and slick eyebrows and, of course, to add clear shine to lips. And finally, save time by choosing eyeshadows with clear glass lids so you can find the one you want without having to rummage through your entire collection.

Once you have identified your beauty 'personality' (see page 10), read the tips below, then make a concerted effort to streamline your make-up kit. Less is definitely more.

If you are a **hoarder**, your make-up bag is probably a minefield, containing umpteen unidentifiable products that are well past their sell-by date. Set yourself a target figure of **ten essential items** to carry around with you and discard the rest.

The **minimalist** is either highly organized or leads such a busy life that she has no time to spend on elaborate make-up. If you fall into this category, make sure the products you own are **multipurpose**. Choose lipsticks that deliver both colour and treatment benefits, and blushers that can also be used as eyeshadows. You'll have much less to carry around.

If the **eclectic** analyses her make-up bag, the chances are that she'll find few of the products in it go together or even suit her. If this sounds like you, treat yourself to a makeover and some expert advice, then make a fresh start and try to build a more **cohesive collection** of cosmetics.

If you are **living in the past**, you've probably been using the same make-up colours for the past ten years, so you, too, will benefit from an in-store makeover and **a new direction**. Look at pictures of models and celebrities in magazines for ideas and inspiration.

Keep it clean

- Hygiene is an important aspect of make-up care. Wash your make-up bag itself every few weeks and rinse brushes, powder puffs and sponges in soapy water at least once a week.
- Cosmetics, like foods, have a limited shelf life, so discard ancient products – most are past their best after six months or so. This is especially true of mascaras and other products that come into contact with the eyes, where risk of infection is high.
- For the same reason, never be tempted to lend or share your make-up.

MEET THE
real BEAUTIES

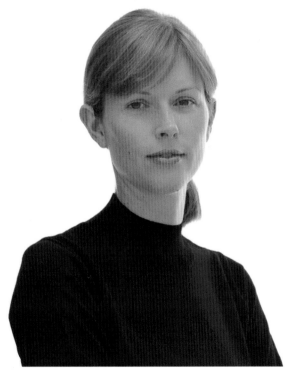
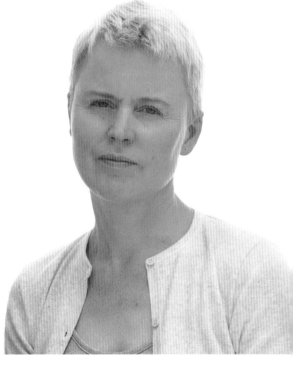

Jo

NORMAL/COMBINATION, FAIR SKIN
FINE, FLYAWAY, FAIR HAIR

Normal skin is usually reasonably plump and a fairly even colour, making it one of the easiest skins to manage. Fine hair is more problematic, but it can be dramatically improved with styling tips and the right products. And fair skin can look wonderful with either subtle or dramatic make-up, as long as the right tones are identified.

Lynne

DRY, MATURE SKIN
GREY HAIR

Mature skins are generally characterized by fine lines and a gradual loss of moisture, firmness and radiance. However, the latest skincare and cosmetic products will give them a new lease of life. And by up-dating their make-up routines, older women can create beautiful, wearable modern looks that will flatter their hair and skin colours.

To ensure Real Beauty **lives up to its name, we have focused on five real women who have had their looks analysed, their make-up routines reassessed and their skin and haircare problems discussed. Each of our five guinea pigs has a specific skin and hair type that presents a different set of problems. Follow their progress through the chapters of the book, paying special attention to the real beauty whose skin and hair type and colouring is closest to your own.**

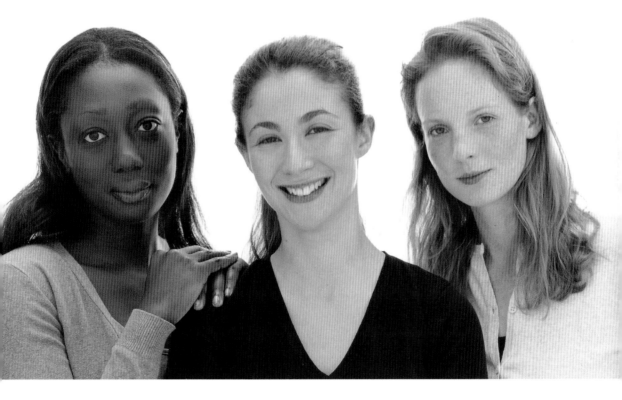

Sandra

DARK SKIN
BLACK HAIR

Dark skins tend to get lumbered with a tough label, which couldn't be further from the truth. Their resilience to the sun does afford some protection, but a gentle skincare regime is still vital. When it comes to make-up, the variety of dark skin tones makes colour selection daunting, but the right texture can make all the difference.

Susanna

OILY, OLIVE SKIN
OILY, LANK, DARK HAIR

Oily skins tend to be thicker than their pale, dry counterparts, and can be prone to enlarged pores and blemishes. On the plus side, they are slightly more resilient and tolerant of the sun, which means they age better. Oil-free make-up will work wonders, and expert advice will help resolve the problems associated with lank, oily hair.

Arabella

PALE, SENSITIVE, FRECKLED SKIN
DRY, FRIZZY, RED HAIR

This very fair, Celtic skin type is, in general, the most sensitive, and women with this colouring are often prone to skin irritation and allergic reactions, as well as being very vulnerable to sun damage. As red hair tends to be dry, it requires special care, while freckly skins usually benefit from some professional make-up tips.

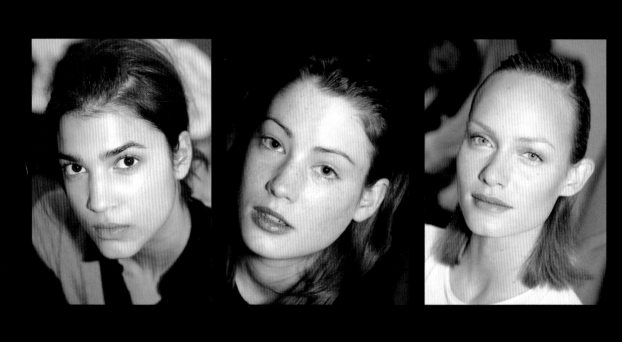

skincare

THE PATH TO
perfect SKIN

Great skin is the basis of great beauty, reflecting youth, vitality and good health. But despite the obvious benefits of a thorough cleansing routine, and the millions of pounds spent each year on creams and lotions, many of us rely on soap and water alone to care for our skin. A little time and effort, however, will improve both its appearance and texture. The first, most important step towards a glowing complexion is identifying

skin helps loosen deep-seated grime and break up stale oil residue.

It is also possible to be overzealous with toners. Wiping the skin until no more grime appears on cotton wool may make us feel deep-cleansed, but it can also remove the skin's protective layer – the stratum corneum – leaving the skin vulnerable to infection. Scruffing, once a popular treat, is now considered too rough for most skins; some therapists believe that sweeping with

Try a gentle routine; it will be kinder to your skin

your skin type correctly (turn to page 14 if you are still unsure). Getting this right will help you to choose products and solutions that are right for you and your skin.

SOFTLY, SOFTLY

Most skincare experts agree that we are often too rough on our skin, scrubbing too hard and using abrasive products that are best left to expert hands. But you can make your routine gentler without reducing its benefits. Warming cleanser in the palms of your hands before applying it helps emulsify the cream, making it more effective. Applying it with your fingertips, rather than cotton wool, can minimize pulling of the skin. And spending a few extra minutes working cleanser into the

a dry cotton-wool ball is enough to remove dead cells from the skin's surface.

Avoid extremes of temperature in your skincare routine as both heat and cold can have adverse effects. Heat can overstimulate the oil-producing sebaceous glands as well as triggering loss of moisture, which results in slacker skin. If you prefer a soap-and-water routine, stick to moderate temperatures, which won't aggravate thread veins or broken capillaries, and mild, specially formulated soaps, which won't upset the skin's natural pH balance. Facial steaming can also be damaging, so try a gentle massage instead – this will deep-cleanse your whole face and relieve the congestion that causes spots (turn to page 54 for a step-by-step guide).

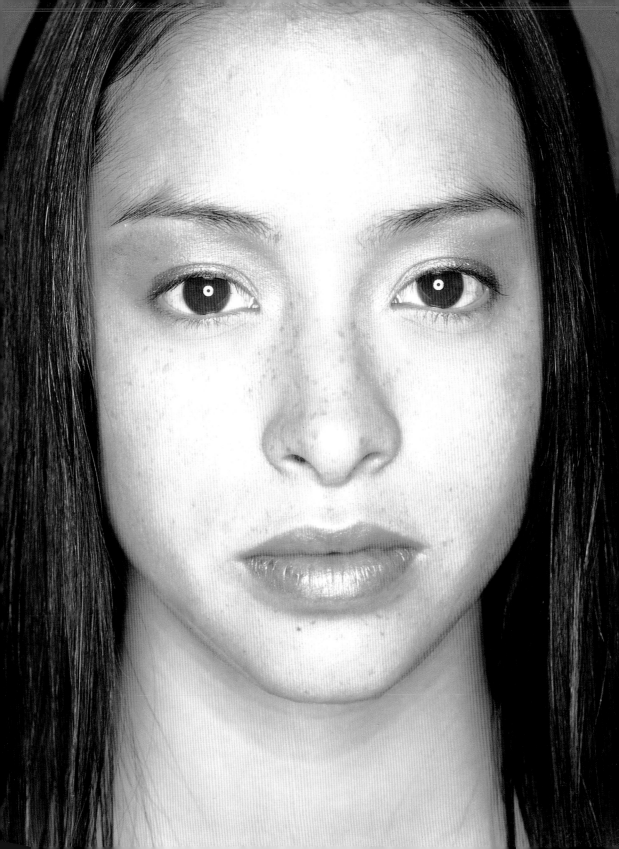

TREAT YOURSELF

A skin-pampering treat is a wonderful way to kickstart a new regime. Skin is a living organ that deserves proper care, and most therapists report a substantial improvement in the texture and condition of the skins they treat. This is partly because an expert eye and a different pair of hands will be able to assess and reach problem areas far more easily than you can yourself – try to practise upward cleansing strokes all over your face and you'll see how difficult it is. And the benefits aren't restricted to your face – an hour with a beauty therapist is a relaxing experience that will relieve stress and give your whole system a boost.

While you are at the salon, make the most of the therapist's expertise and ask questions as she works. Find out what she is doing, which products she feels are right for you and how she would tackle any problems your skin may have. Look out for tips that you can use at home, too. Most therapists remove eye make-up by lightly soaking cotton-wool pads in cool water and a little eye make-up remover, placing them on the eyelids and gently rubbing the pads with the fingertips using a circular motion. This is an effective method that beats rubbing the entire pad over the eye and stretching the skin in the process.

Finally, make a note of how your skin looks and feels at the end of the session, not only as a judge of the facial itself, but as a marker for future improvement.

SPOTS – TO SQUEEZE OR NOT TO SQUEEZE?

Unlike acne spots, most pimples are caused by bacteria invading the skin and causing infections. As the body's white blood cells fight the infection, the spot and

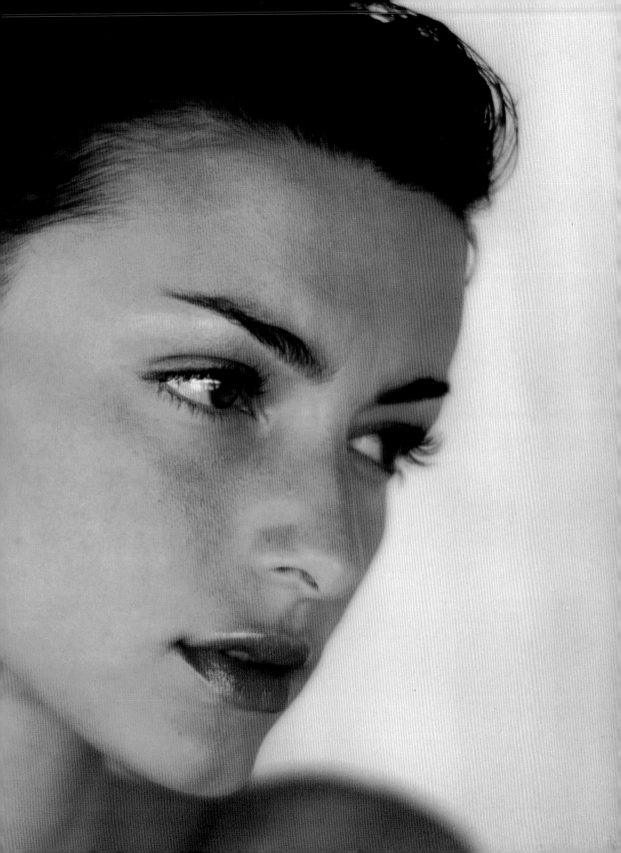

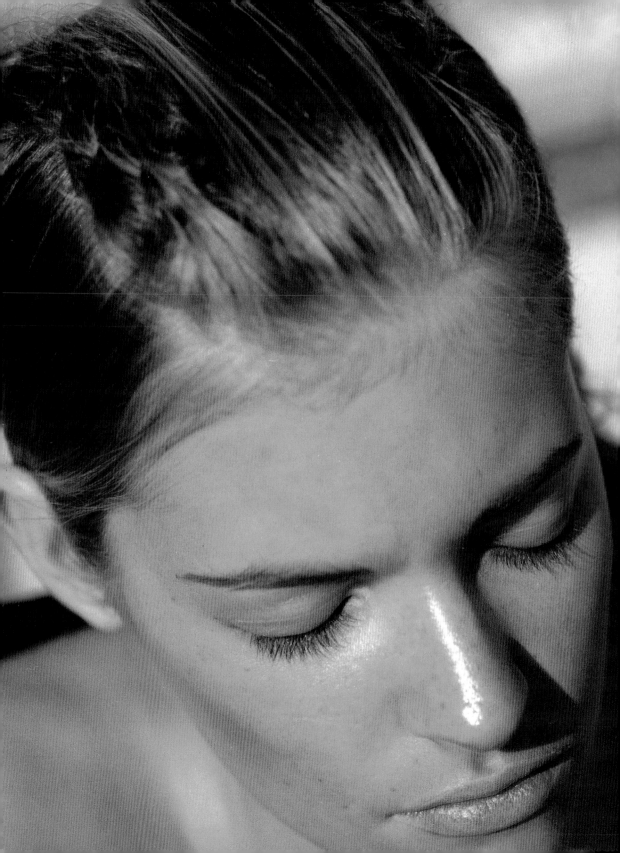

redness surrounding it appears. Squeezing and poking isn't a good idea as you can easily damage pores this way, but if you are going to squeeze, it makes sense to learn a few good practices.

Salons are the best place to observe the art of extraction, by watching a therapist and feeling the pressure applied. At home, make sure you cover your fingertips with tissue before you start and treat the area to a dab of witch hazel or tea tree oil (a powerful natural antiseptic) after squeezing to minimize reinfection. The best time to squeeze spots is at night after a warm bath, when the pores have been lightly steamed and any redness has a chance to subside.

GET GLOWING

Although an effective skincare routine is crucial to a healthy complexion, creams and lotions aren't the only answer. Sleep is a great skin-restorer as cell-renewal processes are activated at night, reaching their peak between 1am and 2am. So while a constant round of parties will eventually take its toll on your skin, a good night's sleep will give its repair mechanisms a chance to kick in and do their stuff.

A brisk, hot shower followed immediately by a blast of cold water is a great quick fix – it has a similar effect to a 15-minute jog, in a fraction of the time. It will rejuvenate your system, boost circulation and energy levels and leave your skin glowing. A walk on the beach, having first applied a protective layer of sunblock, is another option – a dose of oxygen-rich ozone will really pep you up.

Finally, if you want your skin to look better, you have to feel better. Lower stress levels and a positive state of mind are now known to have an impact on the way you look. So while the hormonal changes that are caused by stress can result in spots and blemishes, a happy outlook encourages the production of endorphins, substances that occur naturally in the brain in response to certain triggers. Transmitted around the body via the nervous system, they create a natural high and a feeling of wellbeing. They are also thought to stimulate the body's defences and repair mechanisms, which will have a positive effect on the way you feel and look.

RECIPES FOR SUCCESSFUL SKINCARE

Beauty remedies don't have to be hi-tech and expensive – you can make many of your own using ingredients from your fridge or kitchen cupboard. They're quick and easy to prepare, and even simpler to use.

For a great impurity-removing treatment, take some chilled natural yoghurt and spread it all over your face and neck, as you would a face mask. Leave it for one or two minutes before splashing off with lukewarm water. And for fresh, firm skin in no time at all, whisk an egg white with a little olive oil and apply the mixture to your face, avoiding the eyes and mouth. Leave for ten minutes, then rinse the mixture off with warm water.

Sore eyes can also be soothed with natural ingredients. Chill some full-fat milk in the freezer until it's very cold but not frozen. Then saturate two cotton-wool pads with the milk, place them over your eyes and leave for a couple of minutes. If you suffer from puffy eyes, try pouring boiling water on two camomile teabags. Leave them to cool, then place one over each eye and relax for five minutes.

Simple steps to better skin

- Keep hair off your face with a shower cap or thick towelling band when cleansing.
- Maximize the impact of a face mask by covering your face with a warm towel while the mask is on your skin.
- If you are a soap and water addict, try liquid soap. The emulsifying agents in solid bars are naturally alkaline and can upset your skin's pH balance.
- Always include the entire neck area in your skincare routine. It needs as much care and consideration as your face.
- Rather than steaming your skin, which can be harsh, cover it with a warm towel sprinkled with a few drops of an enlivening essential oil, such as lemon balm or mint, and breathe deeply for a minute or two.

Essential oils

A few carefully chosen essential oils are a welcome addition to any beauty routine. Ready-mixed essential oil-based skincare preparations are available in good health food shops and chemists but, if you prefer, you can buy the oils separately. Only a few essential oils are safe to apply neat – notably, lavender oil. Most must be diluted in a base or carrier oil, and remember to avoid almond or other nut oils if you are allergic to nuts. Some essential oils should be avoided altogether during pregnancy, so check before you buy.

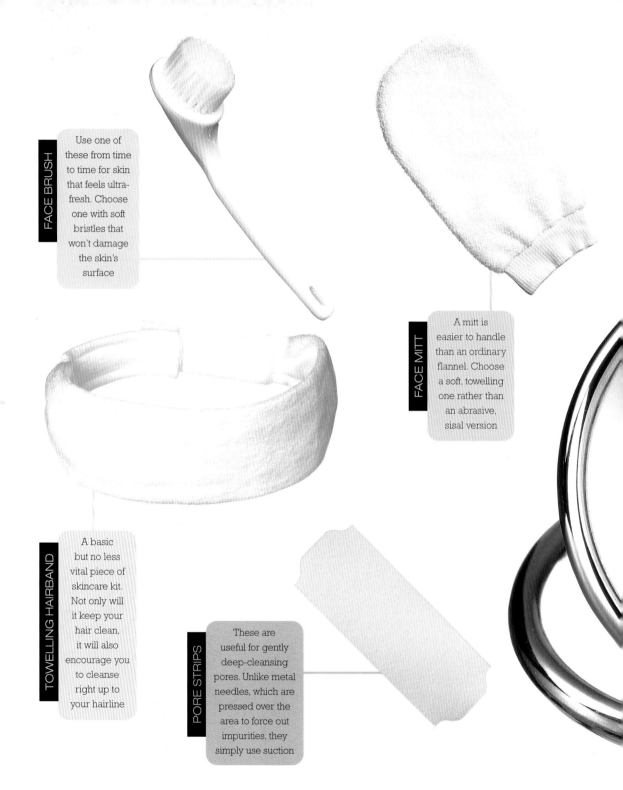

Use one of these from time to time for skin that feels ultra-fresh. Choose one with soft bristles that won't damage the skin's surface

A mitt is easier to handle than an ordinary flannel. Choose a soft, towelling one rather than an abrasive, sisal version

A basic but no less vital piece of skincare kit. Not only will it keep your hair clean, it will also encourage you to cleanse right up to your hairline

These are useful for gently deep-cleansing pores. Unlike metal needles, which are pressed over the area to force out impurities, they simply use suction

know-how

A successful skincare routine depends partly on the right products, but also on a few basic tools. So for skin that's really fresh and clean, invest in this essential cleansing kit

MAGNIFYING MIRROR

These are great for close inspection and care of the skin. Choose one with an in-built stand so both your hands are free

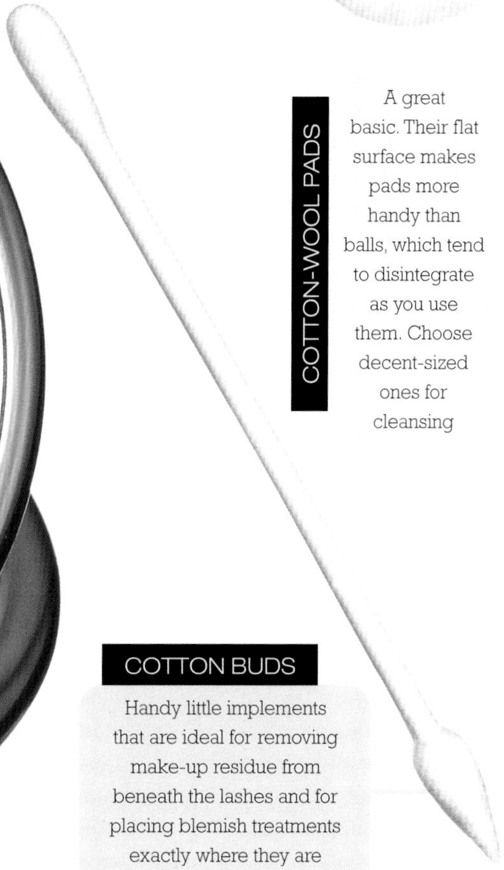

COTTON-WOOL PADS

A great basic. Their flat surface makes pads more handy than balls, which tend to disintegrate as you use them. Choose decent-sized ones for cleansing

COTTON BUDS

Handy little implements that are ideal for removing make-up residue from beneath the lashes and for placing blemish treatments exactly where they are needed

PALE, SENSITIVE, FRECKLED SKIN

see page 21

Because of its sensitive nature, Arabella's skin type needs to be approached with care. A basic **cleanse, tone and moisturize** routine is fine provided it focuses on mild, unfragranced cream or lotion cleansers. Wash-off cleansers may be too harsh or alkaline for this skin type, leaving behind residues that might cause irritation. Toners, too, should only be used if they are alcohol-free and, better still, fragrance-free. The watchword here is **gentleness** and the best routine a simple one.

Sensitive skin tends to be **fine and delicate** so abrasive products such as wash mitts, exfoliating scrubs or enzyme-activated masks should be avoided. Instead, treat yourself to a soothing mask or a **facial massage** that includes a calming essential oil, such as lavender, clary sage or camomile. If you have freckles, don't bleach or scrub at them – they won't go away and trying to get rid of them like this could upset your skin.

avoid

soap and water

highly fragranced products

very astringent products

exfoliating scrubs and masks

look for

soothing ingredients, such as camomile and aloe vera

natural moisturizing ingredients, such as vitamin E

oil-based moisturizers to create a barrier layer

SUN PROFILE

Freckling indicates an uneven distribution of melanin, the skin's natural protective force and the substance that creates the colour associated with tanning. As a result, this type of skin needs extra care and protection in the sun. Look for products containing physical filters, such as titanium dioxide, rather than chemical sunscreens, which sink into your skin and may cause irritation.

AGEING PROFILE

Sensitive skin is more prone to wrinkles and fine lines than the other skin types, due to its fineness and lack of oils. This means that not only should you limit your time in the sun, but you should also shield skin from other environmental hazards, such as cold winds and central heating. Oil-based moisturizers (and most are) will help create a barrier to protect your skin from the elements.

TIP The best buy for this skin is baby cotton wool. Specially formulated for the most delicate of skins, it has none of the microscopic scratchy fibres found in most other cotton wools

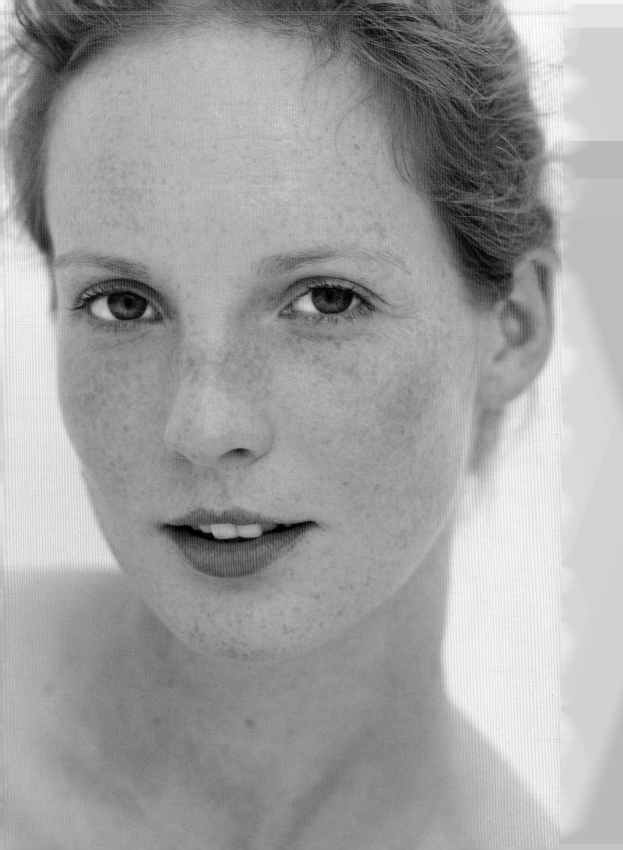

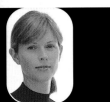
Normal skin like Jo's is fairly easy to care for, so its greatest risk is being taken for granted. Many people confuse combination and normal skins; although normal skin is generally plump and even in colour and tone, it is actually quite common to have the distribution of oil-producing sebaceous glands centred around the nose, chin and forehead, otherwise known as the T-zone. And rather than attempting to split a routine to cover both the oilier parts and the drier cheek areas, this skin type is best treated as a whole.

A wide range of products are suitable for normal/combination skins, so opt for whichever you prefer – mild wash-off cleansers or creamy ones. If you like both, why not use a wash-off cleanser in the mornings for a quick refresher and cream cleanser and toner for a more thorough evening routine. Either way, work from the centre of your face outwards to ensure the areas most likely to attract grime get the most attention.

avoid

harsh products for the T-zone area

exfoliating scrubs

leaving make-up on overnight

strong, alcohol-based toners

look for

nourishing masks as skin treats

moisturizers containing sun protection factors (SPFs)

night creams to make the most of your beauty sleep

SUN PROFILE

A normal skin, especially when it is also fair, lacks the built-in defences of an oilier skin, so good levels of sun protection are essential. Think about incorporating moisturizers and foundations containing sun protection factors (SPFs) into your make-up routine – tinted moisturizers, for example, often contain SPFs. This way you can avoid adding yet another product to your skin.

AGEING PROFILE

If you have normal skin and you care for it well, you will probably begin to notice fine lines in your 30s, and wrinkles and loss of elasticity in your 40s. Sunbathing and smoking will seriously accelerate this process, though, so don't take advantage of your amenable skin type. Its tolerant nature does mean that you should be able to use anti-ageing creams with fairly active ingredients, such as alpha hydroxy acids (AHAs). Off-the-shelf (as opposed to prescribed) vitamin A creams are another option.

TIP Use toner, especially if it is alcohol-based, on pre-dampened cotton-wool pads. This makes it last longer and, more importantly for your skin, makes it milder and less astringent

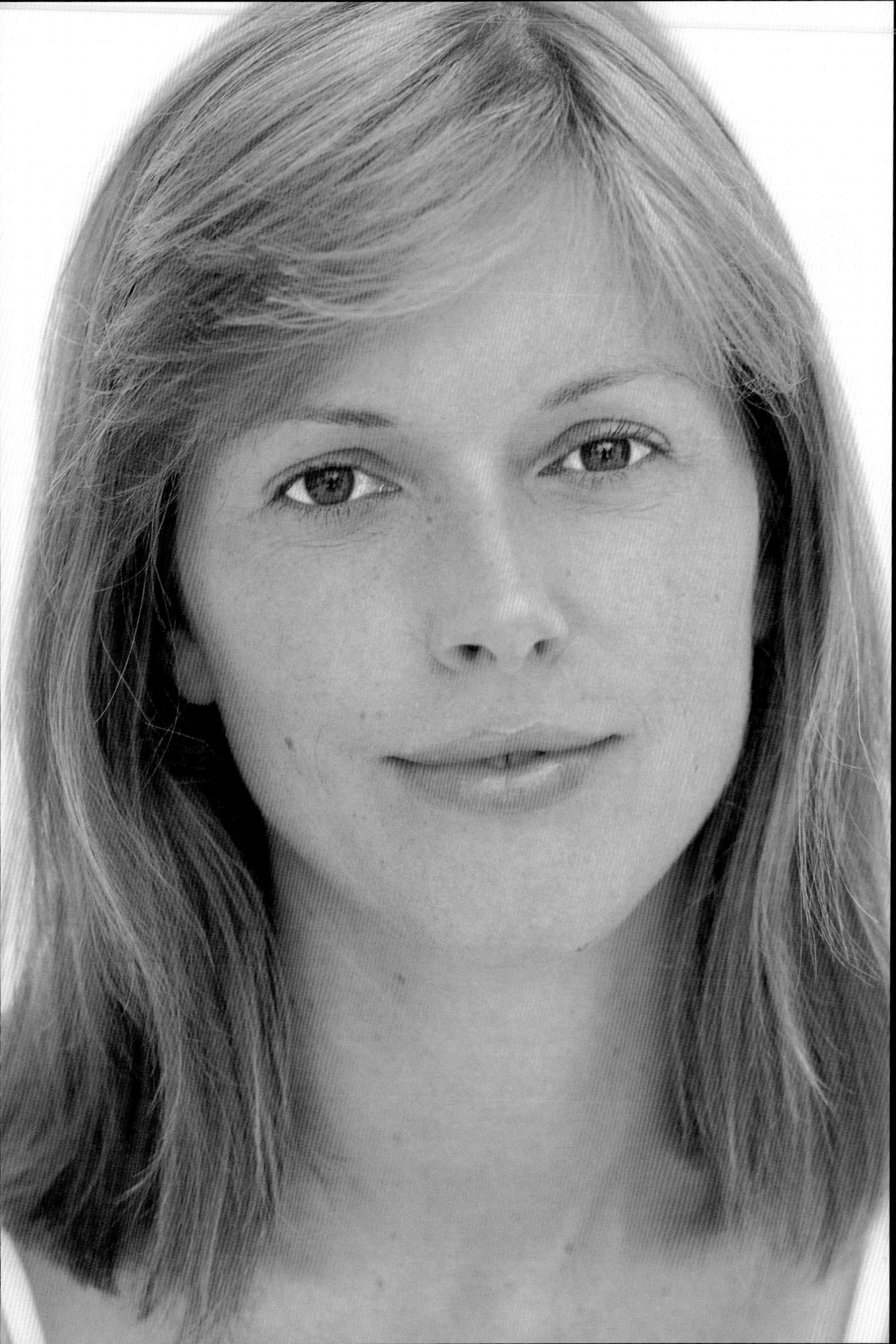

real skin

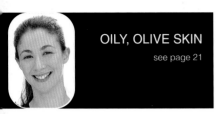

OILY, OLIVE SKIN
see page 21

Oily skin such as Susanna's, in which the sebaceous glands are either more plentiful or more productive than their drier counterparts, is prone to the **harshest treatment**. This is partly because its owners simply believe their skin to be fairly tough, and partly because they often resort to aggressive products to control the excess oil. However, this approach can and does exacerbate the problem.

Instead of soap and water, try a **micro-fine cleansing oil**. Oils actually cling to other oils, so this is more likely to be effective than water, which oils repel. And instead of astringent toners for problem areas, choose milder alternatives. Pore-cleansing strips will suck out dirt, while clay-based masks help remove general grime and excess oils as well as delivering **beneficial minerals** to the skin. Avoid masks that dry completely – stick to those that stay moist. And **don't abandon moisturizers**. Use water-based formulas or those with the words 'oil control' or 'mattifying' on the label.

avoid

soap and water

harsh, alcohol-based toners

oil-based moisturizers

touching your face too much

look for

products labelled non-comedogenic and non-acnegenic

anti-bacterial essential oils, such as tea tree or grapefruit

cleansing oils, rather than rich creams or lotions

SUN PROFILE

This type of skin is slightly less vulnerable to sun damage than its fairer, drier counterparts. Its extra thickness and surface oils provide some protection from the deeper-penetrating rays, and the olive skin tone indicates a more even and plentiful distribution of melanin, the skin's in-built defence system. But these factors are not enough on their own: sun protection should be a feature of any skincare regime.

AGEING PROFILE

Oily skins also tend to age better than dry ones, particularly when they go hand in hand with darker skin tones. But they can still be prone to fine lines, particularly around the mouth and on the forehead. Facial exercises can help counteract these by keeping the muscle structure relaxed and fluid (see page 54 for three quick and easy exercises).

TIP To avoid spreading the bacteria that cause spots, keep your hair tied back and your hands away from your face, and swab your telephone receiver once a week with tea tree oil

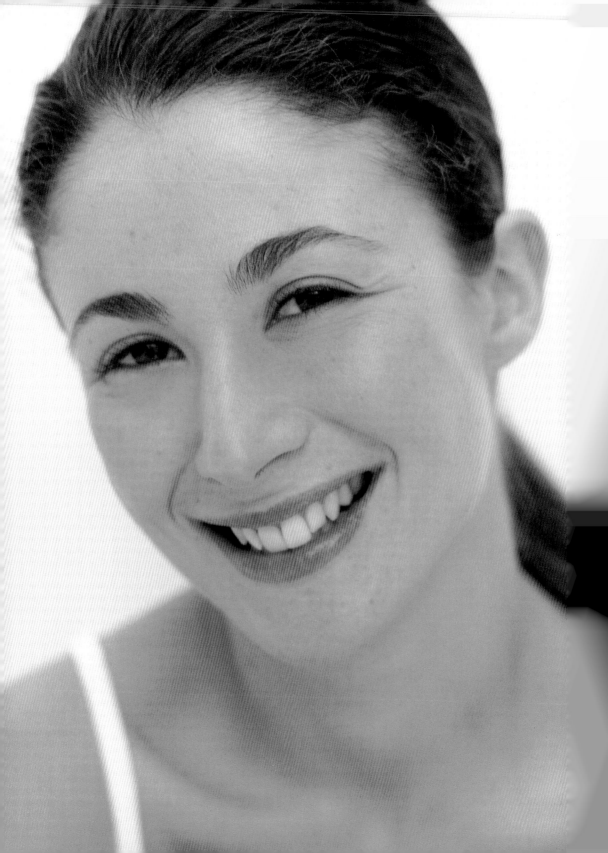

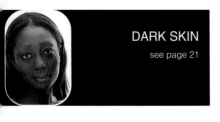

DARK SKIN
see page 21

While there is virtually no difference between the consistency of black and white skins, there is obviously a vast difference in terms of pigment intensity. So while dark skins such as Sandra's tend not to burn in the sun, they are often treated as though they are more resilient than they actually are. In fact, harsh, aggressive products can damage dark skins, making them look patchy and uneven. So avoid abrasive scrubs and exfoliators, as well as products containing active ingredients such as tretinoin and hydrogen peroxide. And handle your skin gently, too – try not to prod or squeeze as this can damage deep tissue layers.

Start your routine with a mild cream cleanser. Then exfoliate with a soft wash mitt or mild toner to remove dead cells, which create a dull, ashy look when left on the skin's surface. Finally, apply moisturizer immediately – it is more effective on new skin cells. For best results, warm it between your fingertips before massaging in.

avoid

products containing tretinoin

skin-bleaching and lightening products

hydrogen peroxide-based skin creams

sisal or scratchy exfoliation pads

look for

micro-bead exfoliators for gentle scruffing

sunscreens that offer both UVA and UVB protection

mild toners containing alpha hydroxy acids (AHAs)

SUN PROFILE

The myth that darker skins do not suffer in the sun is just that. There are about 35 colour divisions in the dark-skin spectrum (as opposed to three in paler skin's) and most of these will tan following sun exposure. So despite dark skin's high levels of melanin, sun protection is still advisable. You can, however, avoid the really high SPFs, and you probably won't need protection all year round.

AGEING PROFILE

Dark skin may not burn in the sun but it is still vulnerable to damage from free radicals, rogue molecules that weaken and destroy skin cells, causing the visible signs of ageing. As the sun triggers free-radical action, use a good sunscreen and invest in products containing the antioxidant vitamins C, E and beta-carotene, nature's antidotes to free-radical damage.

 TIP Dark skins are prone to oiliness, so counter excessive shine with a mattifying, oil-free moisturizer for daily wear

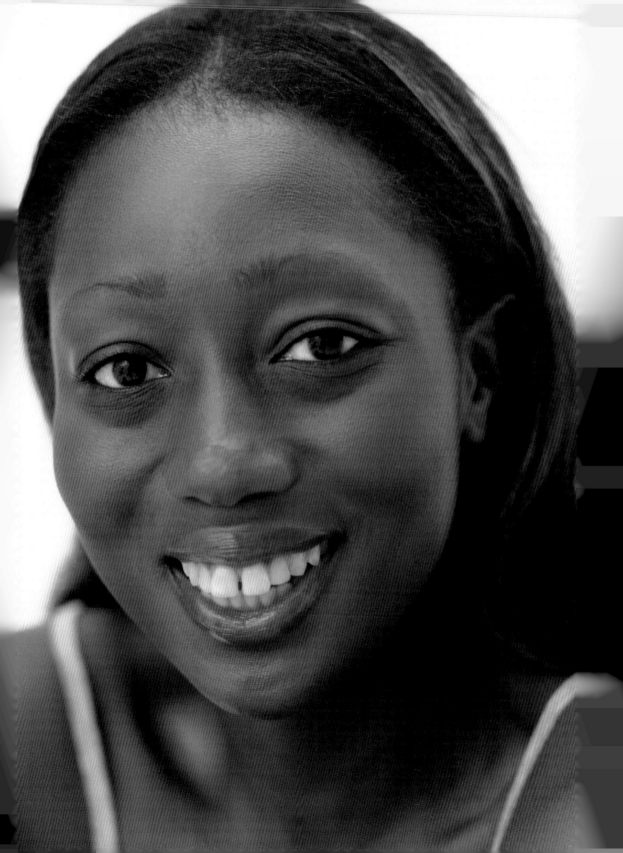

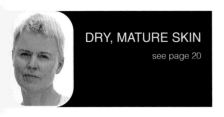
As skin ages, various processes bring about change. The sebaceous glands start to function more slowly, meaning fewer protective oils are produced, and the cells flatten, resulting in greater moisture loss and drier, duller skin. So a routine for a mature skin like Lynne's needs to address a variety of problems. Start with a good cleanser – use a cream or lotion to avoid dehydrating your skin. Wax based cleansers melted between your fingertips will shift any dirt or make-up residue without drying the skin.

Hi-tech moisturizers, such as ceramide creams, are laden with lipids (fats), which are absorbed into the skin, making it feel smoother. Products containing humectants help skin to absorb moisture from the atmosphere, while special treatments, such as essential oil-based preparations, nourishing masks and night creams will also work wonders. In short, your skincare routine should be a layering process, restoring your skin's moisture and oil content with every step.

avoid

lanolin-based creams, which may block pores

very hot or cold water

stress – it always shows up in your skin

look for

humectant ingredients, such as hyaluronic acid

moisturizers containing light-reflecting particles

wax based cleansing products

SUN PROFILE

The sun's damaging action doesn't stop just because your skin has aged a little, and it is never too late to start protecting your skin from its harmful rays. If you already suffer from age spots, try one of the stronger AHA creams, which will diminish them more gently than bleaching.

AGEING PROFILE

A mature skin may lack moisture but, if you choose high-performance hydrating products, it will still reflect light, making it look more youthful and radiant. Choose moisturizers that contain the antioxidant vitamins C, E and beta-carotene to help protect and nourish the skin and enhance production of collagen. This natural material is found in the deeper layers of the skin, where it retains moisture and keeps skin springy.

TIP Plants, particularly umbrella, cheese and spider plants, can help your skin by creating a moisture-rich atmosphere, as well as negating the positive ions emitted by computers

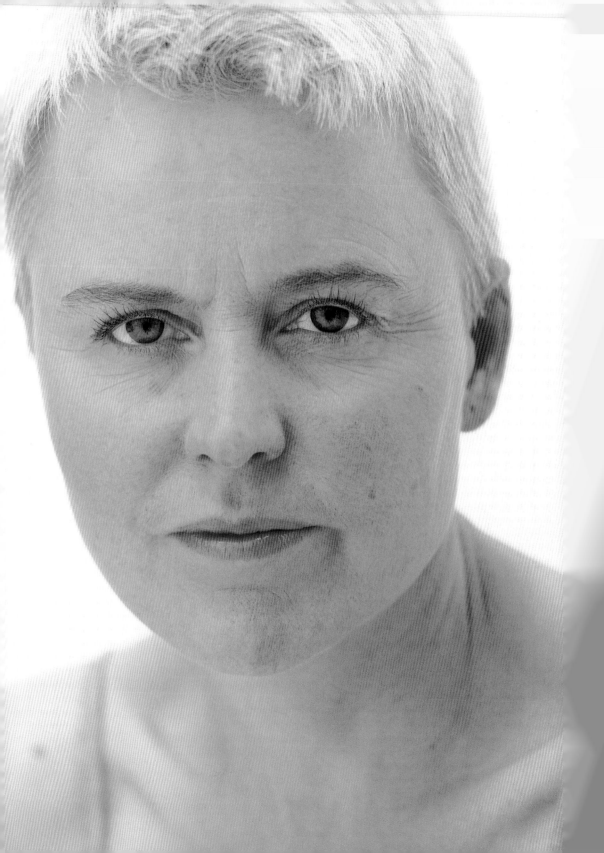

food
FOR THOUGHT

Balance is the key to everything and no more so than in our diets. So while it is impossible for most people to eat freshly prepared foods and straight-from-the-plant fruits and vegetables on a daily basis, it is better to relish each aspect of our diet than to feel guilty about the odd lapse.

Information is what enables us to make the right choices, so learning more about the foods we eat is crucial. It may even throw up a few surprises. Small bottles of freshly squeezed orange juice, for example, may be rich in vitamin C but, because they contain the juice of up to six oranges, they can also be too acidic for sensitive skins. Dairy products, which are undoubtedly essential in moderation, can be tough on the digestive system when consumed in excess, and they are also believed to be a possible cause of allergic reactions. And foods that are rich in iodine, such as eggs, malted breads and shellfish, are thought to trigger acne when eaten in large quantities.

Healthy eating is as much about common sense as anything else. So go easy on hot spices and rich foods, which can be difficult for our digestive systems to cope with, and overprocessed foods, which have little nutritional value. Instead, concentrate on natural, wholesome ingredients and simple cooking methods, such as steaming, grilling and poaching.

Pasta is one of the Western world's staple foodstuffs, providing energy-giving carbohydrates to boost us through our days. Covered in extra virgin olive oil – one of nature's nutritional stars – and served with a crisp, green salad, it makes a deli-

Fresh fruits and vegetables are the key to a healthy diet

cious meal that's low in saturated fats and high in the far healthier monounsaturates. Chocolate, on the other hand, has long been considered one of the skin's worst enemies. And although no one has actually proved that it causes spots, its high fat and refined sugar content means that it is not a great body or skin booster and is more likely to rattle your system than nourish or sustain it.

EATING FOR HEALTH AND VITALITY
Recognizing skin-friendly foods is easy. Antioxidants (principally vitamins C, E and beta-carotene) are acknowledged by nutritionists and skincare experts alike for their health-giving properties. Among other things, they are said to protect against cancer and heart disease, boost the immune system and help delay the visible signs of ageing by neutralizing damaging free radicals. They tend to be found in

yellow, orange and red fruits and veg etables, and dark green, leafy vegetables.

Choose organic produce where pos sible, and steam or eat it raw for maximu flavour and vitamin content. And if yc can't quite manage to get through th

recommended five servings per day, t juicing several fruits each morning for healthy breakfast drink – it will make a gre start to your day.

There are other ways to improve yo diet without giving up your favourite treat High-fibre foods help eliminate toxins, s try replacing white bread, pasta and ric with brown and wild varieties. And re member that alcohol isn't all bad. Organ red wine, for example, has few chemica but is rich in antioxidants, so treat yourse to a glass from time to time. If you car start the day without a shot of caffeine, o for the odd cup of freshly ground coffe rather than several cups of instant. Herb teas and infusions will revive and refres you in place of your usual hot drinks.

And finally, you can never drink tc much water. Six to eight glasses, drur throughout the day, will flush out yo system and keep you hydrated, as well a having a positive effect on your skin.

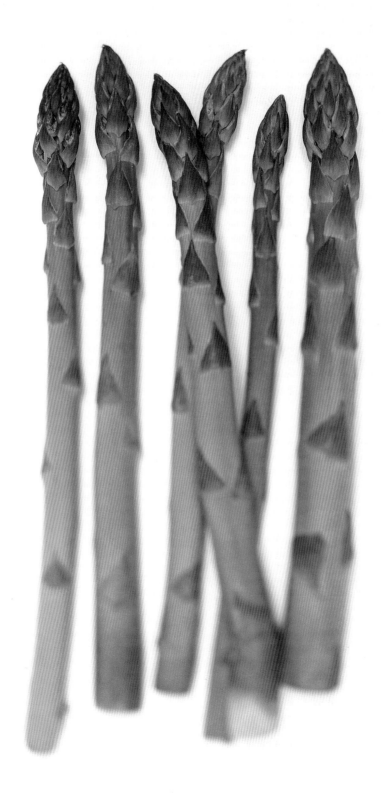

Few foods are wholly good or wholly bad. Those listed below, however, are best eaten in moderation if you suffer from skin or digestive problems. Don't give them up altogether – dairy products, for example, are a good source of calcium and protein, making them a vital part of a balanced diet. Just don't overindulge if you suffer from spots or allergies. Similarly, although many fruits and vegetables are rich in the antioxidant vitamins, which we know are essential for good health, some, such as spinach, are also acidic. This means they are best consumed in small quantities if you have problems with your skin. Boost your vitamin intake with less acidic fruits, such as melon, instead. If you have a skin problem, ideally consult a qualified nutritionist, who will be able to give you advice tailored to your individual needs.

SKIN BADDIES

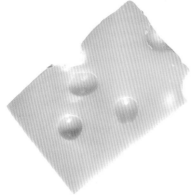

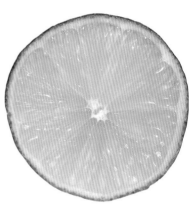

acidic foods

Spinach
Watercress
Sorrel and chard
All citrus fruits
Pineapples
Many berry fruits, including strawberries
Apples and plums
Grapes
Rhubarb
Vinegar and pickled and fermented foods,
    such as sauerkraut
Most alcoholic drinks

dairy foods

Milk
Cream
Hard cheese
Butter
Yoghurt
Ice cream

iodine-rich foods

Sea fish, such as sole, plaice, cod, haddock
Shellfish, such as prawns, oysters, mussels,
    clams, crab, squid
Eggs
Malted breads, wheatgerm
Beer

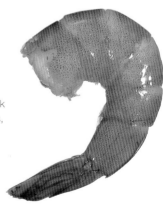

SKIN GOODIES

antioxidant-rich foods

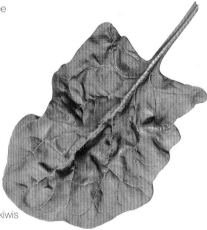

All tomato products, including juice and purée
Onions
Broccoli
Broad beans (fresh and dried)
Brussels sprouts
Spinach
Savoy cabbage
Kale
Spring greens
Red, orange and yellow peppers and chillies
Asparagus
Squash
Sweet potatoes
Avocados
Most fruits, especially mangos, melons and kiwis
Baked beans in tomato sauce
Garlic

purifying foods

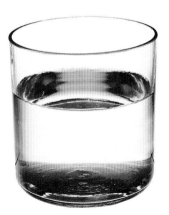

Water
Beetroot
Globe artichokes
Leeks
Cucumber
Onions
Apples
Parsley
Chives
Garlic
Ginger
Chillies
Olive oil

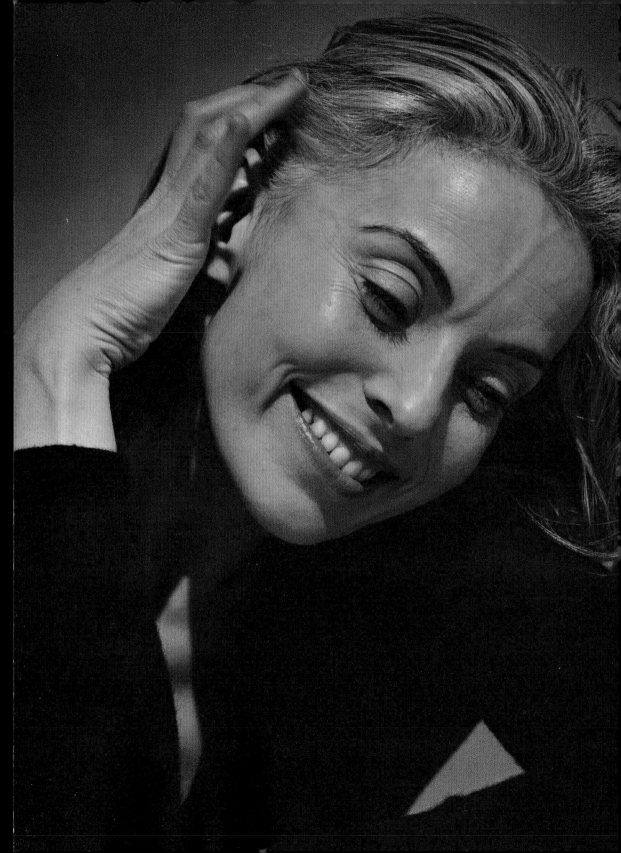

wrinkles
THE GREAT DEBATE

Skin ageing has become one of the obsessions of the late 20th century. As we live longer and women become more prominent in public life, we are bombarded through the media with impossible ideals and images of perfection. But the truth is that skin ageing has very little to do with age itself and plenty to do with environmental factors, genetic predetermination and lifestyle.

Studies estimate that about 80 per cent of skin ageing is caused by over-exposure to the sun. If you have any doubts about the validity of this claim, compare the skin on a part of your body that's rarely exposed to the sun, such as your inner thigh, with the skin on your face and hands. The little-exposed area will hardly show any of the normal signs of ageing – fine lines, wrinkles and lack of firmness – while the exposed areas will have suffered damage at a cellular level, causing the dermis (the skin's deepest layer) to shrink and the surface to shrivel like an old apple.

Even if you think your skin looks fine, don't be complacent. Wrinkles caused by sun damage take ten to 15 years to appear, while estimates suggest that if we avoided exposure to the sun altogether, most of us would retain the complexion of the average 25-year-old.

Sun isn't the only culprit, though. The quality of the air that we breathe is deteriorating, especially in cities, and this too can have a negative impact on our skin. Where we once breathed clean, oxygen-rich air, we now have to cope with high levels of pollution. Ground-level ozone, which is produced when exhaust fumes react with sunlight, triggers skin-agers known as free

A staggering 80% of skin ageing is attributed to sun damage

radicals, which wreak havoc in our bodies and skins.

Oxygen supplies within the skin itself drop as we get older, too. Some figures suggest a gradual decline of up to 70 per cent from the age of 24, which contributes to dull, lifeless, sluggish skin. And while the jury is still out on the oxygen bars that have become so popular in the US, skincare creams containing oxygen seem to be showing good results.

HOLDING BACK THE YEARS
Good bone structure is nature's main weapon in the war against gravity and the inevitable sagging that comes with age. But while we have to make do with what we are born with in this respect, there are some positive steps we can take to minimize the impact of the passage of time. Giving up smoking should be a priority. Not only is it a major cause of facial lines, it also triggers free-radical activity, which we know damages skin.

Sleep is another must for healthy, glowing skin. Make the most of it by applying a light night cream as part of your evening routine and investing in a satin pillowcase to allow your skin to move freely as you sleep. This may seem an odd piece of advice, but dermatologists are able to tell which side we sleep on by looking at pressure lines on the side that's pressed into the pillow and signs of dehydration on the other side. A slippery surface will reduce the risk of skin sticking and dragging.

Finally, a recent study suggested that a positive attitude has a measurable impact on the way we feel about ourselves, which inevitably has a knock-on effect on the way we look – a happy face is usually a radiant and beautiful one. Nearly half of the women questioned felt that a good social life, a wide range of interests and a happy outlook promoted a feeling of health and vitality.

THE SCIENTIFIC APPROACH

The good news is that we don't have to combat the ageing process single-handed – a huge range of skincare products has been developed for this purpose. And although the variety can be confusing, most fall into one of three groups.

Antioxidants The process of ageing is one of cell deterioration and destruction. It sounds grim but it is a natural process, caused in part by the action of free radicals. These rogue molecules, which are triggered by sun-exposure, pollution and smoking, cause many of the visible signs of ageing. But as with every bad guy, there is a good guy, and free radicals' action heroes come in the form of anti-oxidants. Antioxidants are nature's mops, capable of neutralizing free radicals before they do any damage.

The chief antioxidants are vitamin E, vitamin C and beta-carotene, a form of vitamin A. The challenge to skincare companies has not been to identify the benefits of these vitamins, but to find a way of harnessing those benefits. Vitamin C has proved particularly elusive. It is notoriously unstable, breaking down in creams simply because it dissolves in water. But recent breakthroughs have seen it captured in powder form and mixed just before it is used, or shielded by the same elements that preserve it naturally in oranges. Vitamin E is the most commonly found antioxidant.

Alpha hydroxy acids As babies and children, our surface skin cells are renewed every 14 days or so. This is the time it takes cells that are produced deep in the skin to travel to the surface, naturally sloughing the dead cells away in the process. As we age, this rate of renewal slows to around 28 days.

Trying to speed up this cycle to produce more youthful-looking skin is the key to many products, including those that contain alpha hydroxy acids (AHAs). AHAs

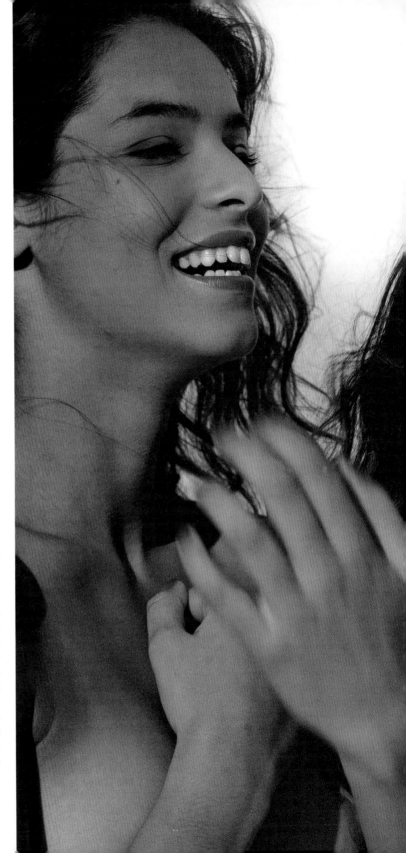

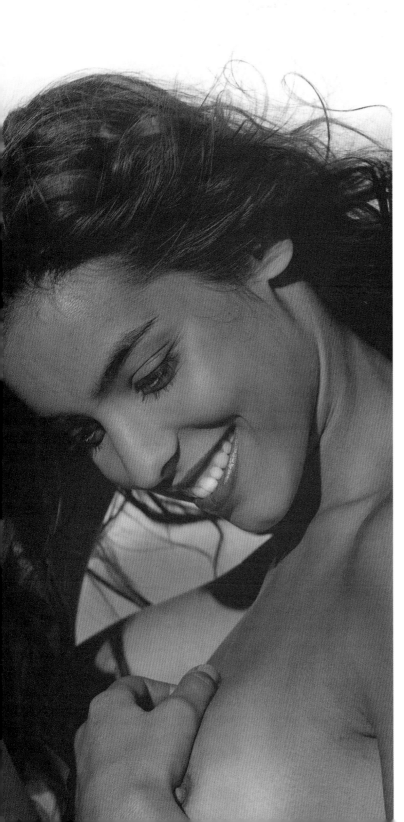

are mild acids derived from natural sources, such as fruits or milk, which help break the bonds of the skin's surface cells, allowing them to be sloughed off. This process triggers the production of new cells, bringing them to the surface more quickly and, in theory, creating plumper, younger-looking skin. However, the acids themselves are now believed to cause skin sensitivities in certain people. It is also thought that the skin may become too accustomed to this chemical sloughing process and lose its natural exfoliating ability. Until the American Food and Drug Administration rules on AHA's, they should be avoided if you have an allergy-prone skin. Other skins should use them as a sporadic revitaliser.

Sunscreens Protecting your skin from the sun is as much a health issue as an anti-ageing one, and sunscreens are now incorporated into a range of cosmetic products as well as sun-protection lotions and creams themselves. Higher sun protection factors (SPFs) provide the best overall cover and, even if your skin doesn't tend to burn, you should choose these rather than the lower factors.

Look for formulations that will protect against UVA and UVB rays (sometimes referred to as broad-spectrum protection). UVA rays penetrate more deeply than UVB and are responsible for the visible signs of ageing, destroying the skin's DNA as well as damaging the elastin and collagen fibres below the surface. Both UVA and UVB rays (which cause sunburn) have now been linked with skin cancer, so it is essential that you are shielded from both.

There's good news for people with sensitive skin. Products containing physical filters, such as titanium dioxide, have been refined and the newest ones contain such finely pulverized particles that they are invisible on your skin. And as they reflect the sun's rays away from the skin, rather than sinking in like chemical sunscreens, they are less likely to irritate.

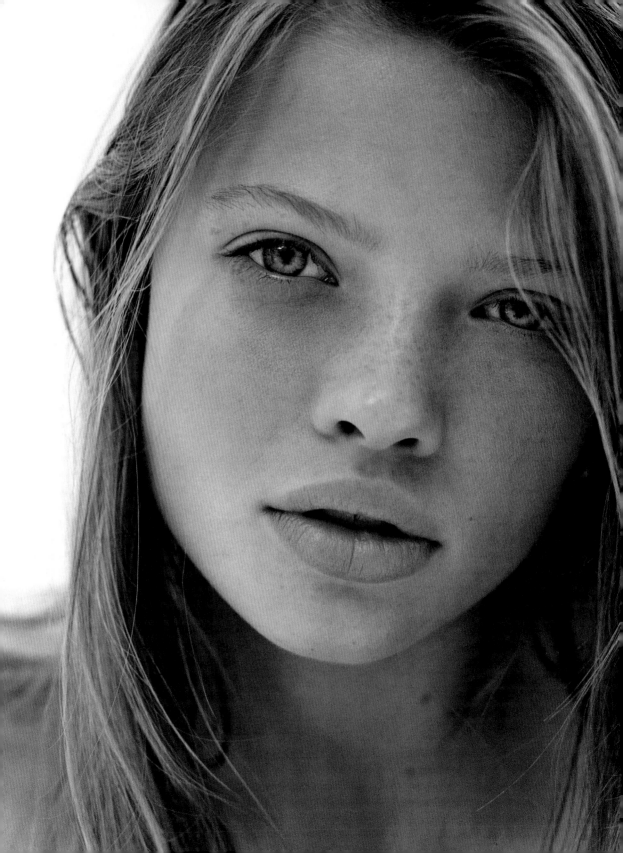

ANTI-AGEING ON PRESCRIPTION

Prescribed anti-wrinkle creams have been dominated by tretinoin, a derivative of vitamin A. Originally developed as an anti-acne treatment, reports that its powerful exfoliating action had a positive effect on wrinkles have made tretinoin a key ingredient in many anti-ageing products. Although low-percentage variations are now available over the counter, the stronger, more effective creams still require referral from a dermatologist.

There are drawbacks. These creams make the skin super-sensitive to UV rays, meaning sun protection is an absolute must. They can also cause uneven pig-mentation, which is likely to be particularly noticeable on dark skins. And as with foods that are rich in vitamin A, they should be avoided by pregnant women.

EYES AND THE AGEING PROCESS

Although a thorough skincare routine should pay equal attention to all areas of the face and neck, it is around the eyes that most of us first notice the signs of ageing. This is partly due to their ex-pressive nature, but also because their constant movement means they suffer more wear and tear than the rest of the face. And to make matters worse, the skin surrounding the eyes is 50 per cent thinner than it is elsewhere on our faces.

Not all the damage that shows up around our eyes is directly related to the ageing process, although it does tend to worsen as we get older. Puffiness in the eye area, for example, is caused by fluid retention, which is often attributed to poor circulation, smoking and alcohol consumption. To combat the problem, try to reassess your lifestyle – a healthy diet and exercise will do more good than excessive amounts of sleep. Derma-tologists recommend sleeping with your head slightly raised so that it is higher than your heart, which will boost lymphatic drainage and help the body to eliminate waste fluids. Puffy-eye sufferers should also try to avoid oily eye creams and rich cleansers, which can exacerbate rather than alleviate the problem.

Dark circles are another case in point. They can be hereditary but they can also indicate a build-up of toxins or a simple lack of sleep. But whatever their cause, the result is a tired, old-looking face. In some ways, this is the easiest problem to rectify as dark circles can be quickly and easily disguised with make-up. For a longer-term solution, you could try a gentle eye-massage exercise to boost the circ-ulation in the eye area (see page 54 for a step-by-step guide to facial massage).

Under-eye bags occur when the fatty tissue that's stored naturally under the eye is damaged or deteriorates with age. This problem can be made worse by rough treatment when cleansing, applying make-up or simply by rubbing the eyes too vigorously. Try to be gentle when applying eye creams: use light tapping movements to deposit the cream gently around the eye area and never, ever drag the skin.

Crows' feet, the ultimate ageing sign, are the facial lines we really love to hate. Most have been caused by simple repetition of the same expression, and that expression is usually smiling. So apart from trying to avoid squinting and applying sun-protection products, just think posi-tively and rename them laughter lines.

Testing, testing…

You've identified your skin type and chosen the products you need, but how can you be sure that they'll work? Sadly, there are no guarantees of success, but what we do know is that all cosmetics are tested in one or more of the following ways before they go on sale:

- In a skin biopsy, slivers of skin are treated with the product in question, and then examined under a microscope for any plumping or refining changes.
- Replica skin cells, which imitate human skin, are cultured in laboratory conditions, and used to test products.
- A cutometer, a device used to measure skin elasticity, is useful for assessing products during the course of a trial. It literally pulls and releases the skin, timing the 'bounce'. The faster this 'bounce', the more elastic the skin.
- A chroma strip is applied like sticky tape and pulled away from the skin. The cell debris left behind can be measured to assess a product's exfoliating potential.
- Image analysis, in which a scanning device transmits a three-dimensional image of the skin's surface to a computer, is useful to show changes in the skin during product trials.
- Silicone imprints work in a similar way. These rubbery imprints can be taken from the skin over a period of time, leaving a detailed impression of its surface condition, and any changes.

It is worth remembering that products do tend to perform better in trials than they do at home, probably because testers follow extremely strict routines, while we are often less thorough in the privacy of our own bathrooms. There's no doubt that a disciplined regime will pay dividends.

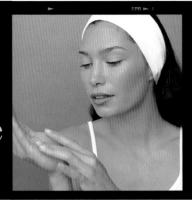
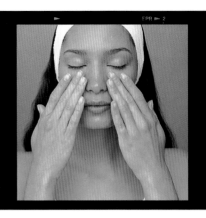

HOW TO
salon-cleanse
at home

One of the keys to beautiful skin is a cleansing routine that's gentle, thorough and relaxing

1 Take a clean towelling headband, then gather your hair back and secure it away from your face. Squeeze a walnut-sized blob of cleanser into your palm and gently warm it between your hands.

2 Apply the cleanser with your fingertips, beginning in the centre of your face and working upwards and outwards to make sure you get under the very fine hairs that cover your face. Tissue off any excess cleanser.

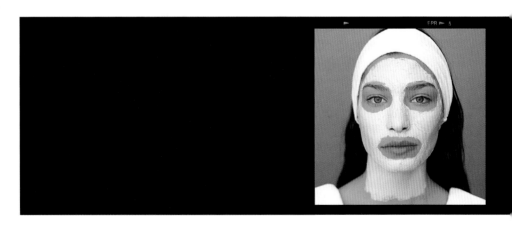

5 Apply a face mask, taking care to avoid the eye and mouth area. Don't forget your neck, which should be treated to each step in the cleansing routine. Tuck tissues into the neckline of your robe or top to protect it from the mask.

masterclass

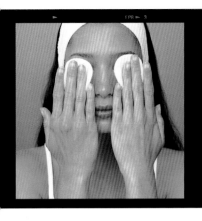

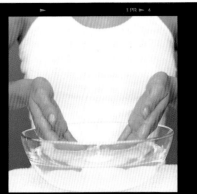

Soak two cotton-wool pads in cool water and then douse them in make-up remover. Lay one over each eye, wait for a few seconds, then rub your fingertips lightly over the surface of the pads to remove any traces of eye make-up.

Using clean cotton-wool pads soaked in warm water and alcohol-free toner, sweep the rest of your face to remove the cleanser. Then gently splash with cool water to stimulate the skin before applying a face mask.

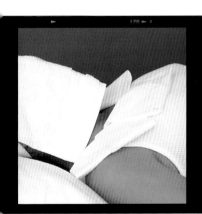

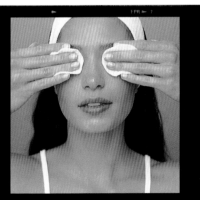

Take a warm towel and sprinkle it with a couple of drops of a relaxing essential oil, such as lavender, camomile or clary sage. Lie back, place the towel over your face and relax for ten minutes to allow the mask's nutrients to penetrate your skin.

Tissue the mask off gently and then, using clean cotton-wool pads soaked in warm water, remove any remaining traces. Finish by soaking two more pads in cold water and place one over each eye. Leave for a few seconds to cool and invigorate you.

HOW TO
massage
your face

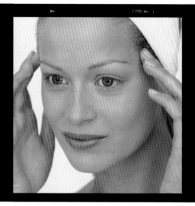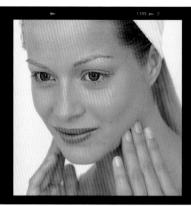

Pamper your skin and give your whole system a boost with a stress-relieving massage

1 Coat your fingertips with a massage oil (blended with a couple of drops of essential oil if you wish). Using light, circular movements, work from the centre of your forehead out to your temples. Repeat across your cheekbones and out to your ears, tugging gently at the lobes. Do the same across your jawline.

2 Using light, tapping movements, take your fingertips along the jawline again, beginning in the centre and working out. This helps boost lymphatic drainage in this area, which is prone to congestion and tension.

HOW TO
exercise
your face

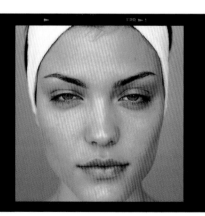

Keep the muscles of your face and neck in tip-top condition with these easy exercises

1 Stand in front of a mirror, look straight ahead at your eyes and slowly narrow them. You will feel a slight tightening under each eye as the muscle contracts inwards. Repeat five times, holding the position for a few seconds each time.

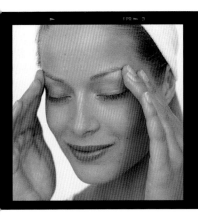

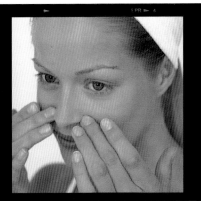

3 Now, using two fingertips and light, pressing movements, work around the inner edges of your eye sockets. Press only as hard as is comfortable and concentrate on the bony area, rather than the eye or lid.

4 Finally, place two fingertips either side of your nose and, using small pressing movements, move down from the nostrils. Work out in a diagonal line, finishing at the corners of your mouth.

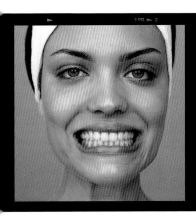

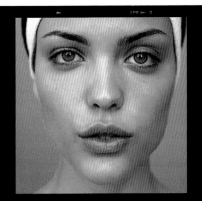

2 The jaw clencher looks like an extreme grimace and you should be able to feel the muscles tense and relax all the way down your neck as you hold and release the position. Repeat four or five times, holding for a couple of seconds each time.

3 This is what top models do to help relax the mouth and ease expression and tension lines. Simply let your mouth area slacken, then blow gently through your lips. Don't overinflate your cheeks – the idea is simply to blow lightly. Repeat a couple of times.

masterclass

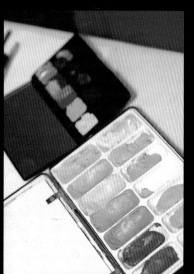
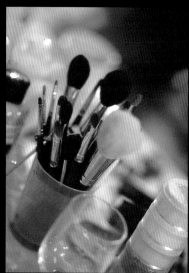
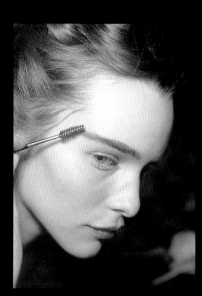

make-up
basics

YOUR BEST
base EVER

Your skincare routine doesn't stop with cleansing, toning and moisturizing. While this cleans and nourishes your skin, a base can give it the final finish, ironing out imperfections and creating an even skin tone.

Make-up also creates an effective barrier between your skin and the elements. The pigments and moisturizers in many modern base products will keep your skin soft and supple as well as protecting it from the damaging effects of the environment, and many foundations contain skin-nourishing extras such as vitamin E, which will continue the good work of your skincare regime.

Whether you choose a fluid, compact or solid-stick foundation, it will probably contain sun protection factors that will reinforce the protection offered by the pigment particles themselves. Check the label to see what level of protection yours provides, and if it doesn't contain SPFs, make sure you apply a separate sunscreen under your make-up. Don't try to save money by using the same product on your face and body – a sunscreen that has been designed specifically for the face will be lighter and less oily, which means it will look better on your skin.

Pre-base products will provide a great surface for colour application, especially if you suffer from oily skin. They are usually creamy gel formulas, and should be applied over moisturizer rather than in its place. Search out primers or moisturizers that have been designed to go under base products; they will help your foundation or powder adhere to the skin so it won't slip and slide over your face or go cloggy as the day progresses.

There is also a growing selection of products for dark skins; great shades and effective formulations with higher pigment levels will prevent your base from looking chalky or ashy. So if you've never worn base before, why not pick up a sample and see what a difference it can make?

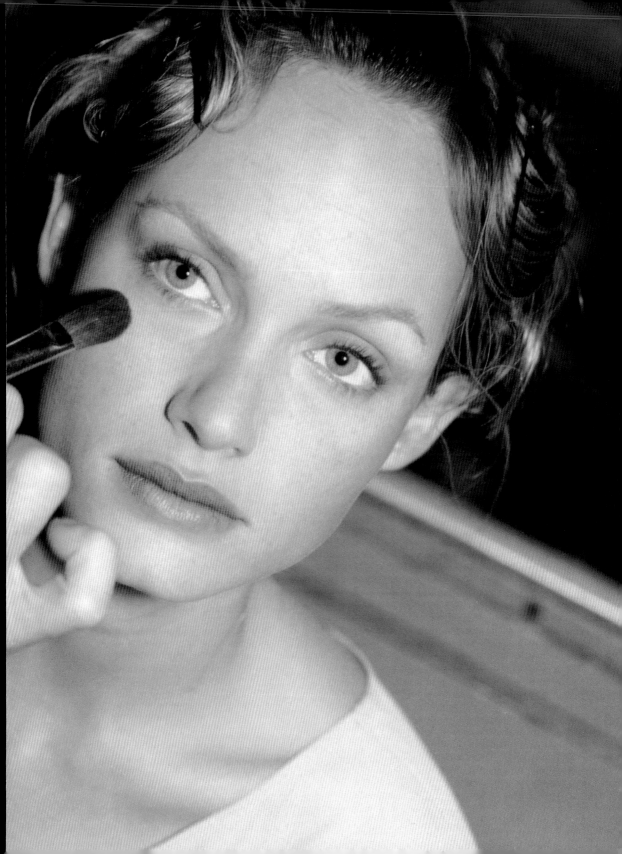

Most of us assume concealers are designed purely for under-eye shadows or blemishes. In fact, when they are properly used they can lift weary lines from other areas of the face and rectify the shadowy grey areas that appear when the skin sags as we age. The natural indents running from the side of the nostrils to the corner of the mouth, for example, are classic age giveaways that can easily be masked. Don't use an ultra-pale concealer on this area – it will be very noticeable, which is the one thing concealer shouldn't be. Choose one that's slightly warmer than the shade you would normally use, or dab on a slightly lighter shade of your regular foundation.

Concealers are technical tools that vary in weight and purpose. A common mistake is to believe that one product will meet all your needs, which is rarely the case. Most of us need two types of concealer, a fine, light-reflective one to deal with shadows, and a denser block to cover blemishes. For a step-by-step guide to using both effectively, turn to page 78.

concealer

Peachy or slightly yellow-toned concealers are best for covering under-eye shadows as they help redress the blue-grey tinge of dark circles. Pinky-toned concealers are simply too cool and will only emphasize the greyish colour. Modern formulations often contain light-reflective pigments that bounce light away from the skin to plump out shadowy areas, so watch where you apply them. Be careful not to cover the eye bag itself, as you may actually draw attention to it. These concealers aren't suitable for covering bumps and blemishes.

Never use a very pale concealer right up to the lower lashes as it can actually make your eyes look smaller. Instead, blend it upwards and fade it out very carefully before you reach the lashes.

Use a flat, sable brush to help direct concealer over thread veins and broken capillaries and apply it over rather than under your foundation. This way you will only need to cover the veins that are visible through the foundation rather than the whole lot.

If you suffer from red patches, look for one of the ranges that includes greenish-tinted concealers. These tone down redness, but they should be used with real lightness and care.

Choose a cream, compact or solid stick for covering spots. Rich in pigment and powder particles, these formulations provide intense coverage, making them unsuitable for use under the eyes or for other shadowy areas. Look for spot cover-ups that contain active healing ingredients, such as arnica, tea tree or clary sage, to treat as well as hide blemishes. And always use a small brush to apply spot concealers. You can be more precise and, by regularly cleaning the brush, will avoid spreading bacteria from your skin to the concealer.

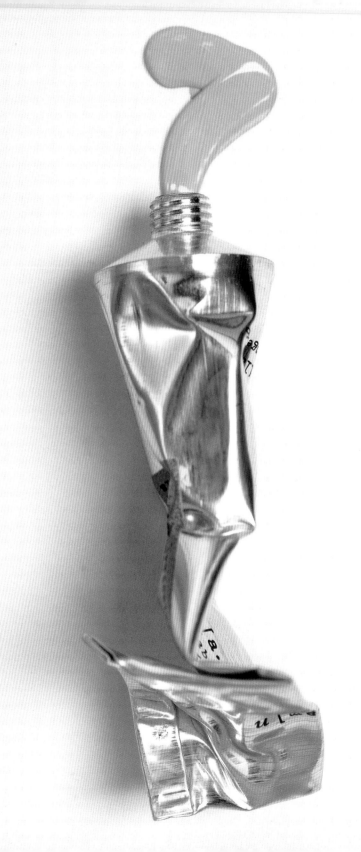

foundation

Select a foundation that matches your skin tone exactly. Never go for a darker shade in the hope that it will make you look more tanned and healthy. It's one thing to wear a tinted moisturiser, which is light and sheer, but the heavier texture of most foundations will be far more obvious. Not only will a darker shade look unnatural, it will also be almost impossible to blend at the edges.

Update your foundation seasonally. What looked right as a make-up base in mid-winter may look a little pale and ghostly come the summer months, when you'll probably want a lighter texture and subtler shade.

Experiment with the iridescent versions now available, but keep them for evening wear. Their pearlized sheen is too glitzy and shiny for use during the day, and may even highlight fine lines and wrinkles that would be invisible in evening light.

Throw out old foundations. Like all cosmetics, they have a limited shelf life and if the oil and pigment parts have started to separate, they are almost certainly past their sell-by date.

Choose your foundation according to its coverage as well as its shade. Sheer formulations are great for youthful skins and flawless complexions, but for more complete coverage, opt for a cream or compact foundation.

Foundation has been transformed from the orange gloop of the past into one of the face's modern miracle workers, giving stressed skins a virtually undetectable helping hand. The breakthrough for most formulations came with the introduction of volatile silicones, microscopic ingredients that give modern base products great 'slip' or spreadability. Once the foundation is applied, they evaporate, leaving a smooth, semi-matt finish.

As with many great make-up inventions, knowing how to use these products is crucial. The evaporation process means they dry more rapidly than their oilier counterparts, which means you have less time to work them over your skin. The heat of your fingertips can also make the silicones evaporate so it's best to use a sponge chip, which will help spread the foundation quickly. This may sound daunting but it produces such a natural finish that it's worth persevering with the technique (turn to page 80 for a step-by-step guide).

The other good news for foundation was the introduction of light-reflecting pigments. These cause light to be bounced away from the skin's surface, making it look younger and smoother. To appreciate the effect, apply foundation to one side of your face and look in the mirror. The foundation should add luminosity to tired skin and throw fine lines into soft focus. Another bonus is the fact that it will make your skin look as good in artificial light as it does in natural light. Smaller, more rounded pigment particles are another feature of good, modern foundations. They are less likely to clump together, which means they create a more even skin tone.

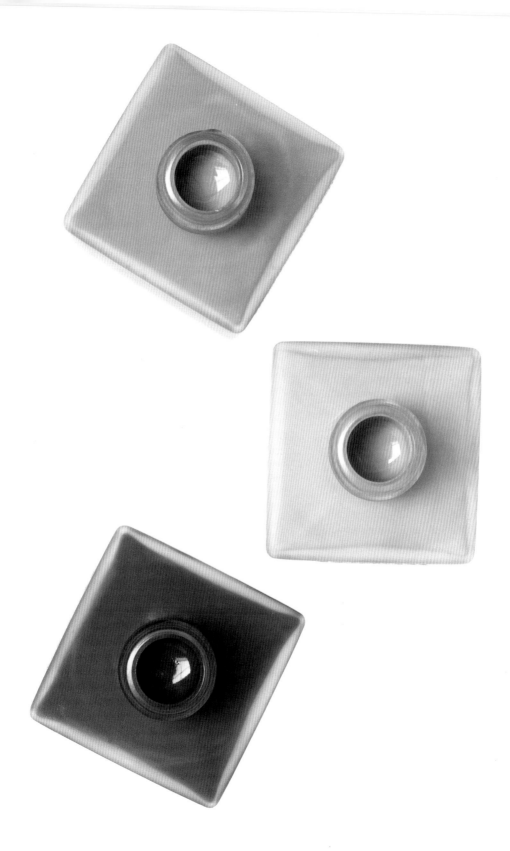

Like foundation, powder has been transformed by scientific advances and is no longer the cakey product it once was. Featherlight loose powder, once the sole preserve of make-up artists, is now a key element of any self-respecting make-up kit. The shade selection has moved on, too. Powder used to come in almost every shade of pink – the so-called flesh tones – but it is now available in a much wider range of yellow-toned banana and cream hues. These are the colours preferred by make-up artists, who know that most skins aren't actually pink and that pinky tones can accentuate dull, grey shadows.

Although powder can be applied on its own over nude skin, it is really a finishing product that's best used to create an invisible, mattifying layer over foundation. If you do want to use it directly on your skin, make sure your moisturizer has been thoroughly absorbed. Modern powders are also sheer enough to apply over the eyelids, but if you want to try this, use a slightly smaller brush.

Loose powder wins hands down over the compressed variety, which has to be applied with a powder puff. The puffs often pick up too much powder, which makes it all too easy to remove the foundation you've carefully applied, or to deliver too much powder to a particular area. Another problem is that powder puffs transfer skin and foundation oils back on to the surface of the compact, sealing the powder and making it virtually impossible to pick up on the puff the next time. Loose powder, although a little messier, is designed to be picked up on a brush that can then be shaken to remove any excess before it touches your face (see page 80 for a foolproof guide to powder application).

Don't wear too much powder during the day, whatever your skin type. Not only will it make your make-up base look obvious, but it may also have a drying effect on your skin.

Decant a little loose powder into a small, transparent, screw-top pot to carry around, rather than keeping a large one in your make-up bag. It will be lighter and there'll be less chance of a spillage.

When applying powder, centre a loaded brush in the middle of your face and work outwards. This way, the shiniest areas get the heaviest delivery of product. If crows' feet are a problem, avoid the area around your eyes as powder may make them more noticeable.

If you do overdo your powder application, skim over your face with a clean powder brush, or lightly roll a fresh ball of cotton wool over the surface of your skin to remove the excess.

Buy powder that matches your foundation colour exactly and never be tempted to try a darker powder shade over your base. You can work the other way around, though, for a flattering evening look. Choose a foundation that's slightly darker than your normal one and dust paler powder over the top. This gives extra depth and creates an illusion of slightly plumper skin.

powder

blusher

Blusher is one of those joyous cosmetics that can revamp a tired face in seconds, creating a youthful, healthy glow and enhancing shy and retiring cheekbones. Used correctly, it is as indispensable as concealer but most of us approach it with trepidation, remembering the streaky results or overcoloured cheeks of our youth. Modern formulations, however, are much easier to apply and blend, even if you've chosen a strong colour. And if you do make a mistake, simply sweep translucent powder over the cheek area to tone it down.

The trickiest thing with blusher is choosing the right formulation. Follow the make-up artists' golden rule and apply like over like. If you've used face powder, use powder blush; on foundation, opt for cream blush and on bare, moisturized skin, try gel blush. Follow the tips below for easy application.

Sculpting the face using blusher should only be attempted when you feel confident with your blusher, and it's a good idea to practise the technique a few times before you face the world. Choose a neutral shade that's slightly darker than your usual foundation – pinky tones are more suitable for emphasizing the voluptuous parts of the face than for this sculpted look.

To shade under and enhance the cheekbones, take your darker shade and work in upturned crescent movements just at the cheek hollow (to find your cheek hollow, suck in your cheeks – the resulting concave areas should show you where to apply the colour). Complete the effect by sweeping highlighter over the very outer demarcation of your cheekbones, just below and beyond your eyes. Remember to blend well to avoid harsh lines, and don't take the shader colour too far into the centre of your face.

The halo glow is a wonderful trick for highlighting the forehead area and giving it a childlike, domed appearance – simply dust a little golden blusher or powder just around the hairline. A nip of golden shadow under the tip of the nose also gives it a lift. You can brush a little powder under your chin for added definition to the jaw area, but be careful not to overdo it – this is a difficult area to judge.

Powder blush Once you have loaded a blusher brush with powder colour, brush it over the back of your hand a couple of times to get rid of any excess. Then work from the centre of your cheeks out to the edges – this is because most peachy-pink shades should be used to play up the apples or domes of the cheeks. And to avoid a stripy look, work the blusher brush in generous circular movements.

Cream blush Modern cream blushers have been injected with so much easy spreadability that you only need to start with a little on your fingertips. Apply straight to your face and build the colour gradually rather than overplaying it initially – it's much easier to add than to take away. Start working over the cheekbones, blending the colour downwards and outwards to avoid an obvious cut-off line.

Gel blush The new gel blushers are great for applying directly to moisturized or nude skin, which makes them perfect for a quick burst of colour. Make sure you start from the middle of your cheeks and blend outwards so the colour doesn't look too intense at the hairline. Gels are ideal for a youthful, glowing look so concentrate them on the appley or central round of the cheek itself.

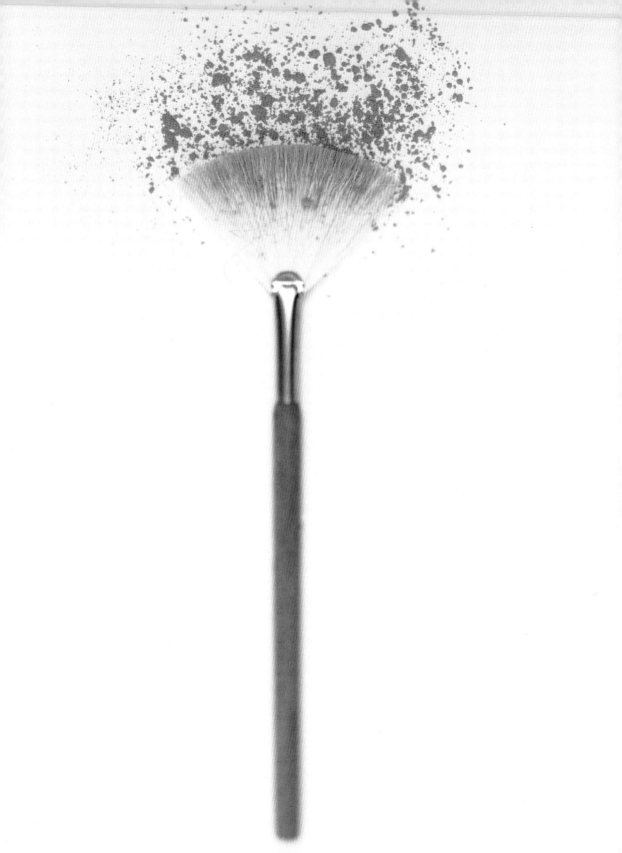

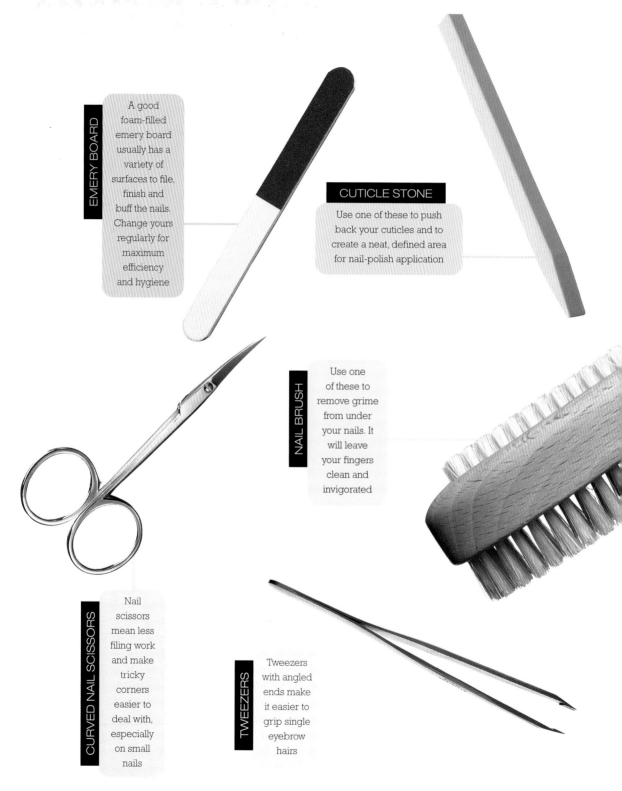

A good foam-filled emery board usually has a variety of surfaces to file, finish and buff the nails. Change yours regularly for maximum efficiency and hygiene

CUTICLE STONE

Use one of these to push back your cuticles and to create a neat, defined area for nail-polish application

NAIL BRUSH

Use one of these to remove grime from under your nails. It will leave your fingers clean and invigorated

CURVED NAIL SCISSORS

Nail scissors mean less filing work and make tricky corners easier to deal with, especially on small nails

TWEEZERS

Tweezers with angled ends make it easier to grip single eyebrow hairs

You'll never have perfect brows, nails or lashes without the right equipment, so take a look at the simple, inexpensive tools on these pages and fill in the gaps in your collection

FACE PAPERS

These can help absorb unwanted oils from the skin's surface on stressful days, so you won't have to resort to more powder. And they're easier to carry around

SHARPENER

A sharpener will keep your make-up pencils in shape. Clean the insides regularly with a cotton bud, or colour residue will muddy fresh pencils

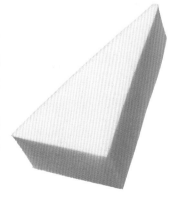

EYELASH CURLERS

Metal curlers are better than plastic ones. They create a better curl and won't damage the eyelashes unless you yank them

SPONGE CHIPS

Dense, foam sponges are great for applying foundation. Rinse them regularly in a little gel cleanser and water

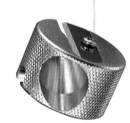

BEAUTIFUL
brows

Slick alternatives to plucking your brows

- Combing your brows with a dense-bristled eyebrow brush will help define them. Some make-up artists use toothbrush heads to do this if the bristles are set very close together.

- For a glossy finish, apply either a little eyebrow gel or petroleum jelly to the brush before you use it. Always brush eyebrows up slightly and then along, to neaten any spiky hairs.

- To hold your brows in place securely, you can spray a little hairspray on to the brush before you use it. This will create a really neat finish.

E yebrows are one of our most defining features. They frame our eyes and mark the horizontal planes dividing the face into its three main sections: forehead, cheeks and mouth. Neat, tidy eyebrows can make a drastic difference to our overall appearance, so their grooming should be high on our list of beauty priorities.

The general aim of home eyebrow-plucking should be to tidy and lightly shape the brows rather than to alter their shape radically. Resist the temptation to overpluck as this can leave you with a permanently startled expression. Worse still, it can hamper the future growth of your brows. It's fine to pluck the odd stray hair from above the brows, but most beauty therapists recommend that you concentrate on those beneath the brow.

Remember that your main objective when tweezing is to open up the eye area. Plucking from beneath the brow will increase the space between the brow and the eye itself, creating an illusion of larger eyes while defining the browbone. Lightly tidying the area above the bridge of the nose is also a good idea but, again, don't overdo it and take the starting point of your eyebrows too far back. This will only appear to widen the bridge of your nose.

If you are really sensitive to pain, numb the brow area with an ice cube before you start to pluck. Alternatively, take your cue from top make-up artists, who recommend either a dab of clove oil or a smear of baby teething gel to deaden pain. And to check whether you are better off without specific hairs, hold them between the tweezers away from the brow before you pluck.

CHOOSING THE RIGHT PENCIL

Eyebrow pencils used to come in just two shades, black and dark brown, both of which were too dark for the average brow. Dark colours can make the brows look false and, while this may work for a dramatic evening look, it is too heavy for day-to-day definition. As a rule, our eyebrows tend to be a little lighter than our hair colour. This fact has at last been recognized by the beauty houses, and most now provide a good selection of tawny and light brown shades. Some even offer very pale fawn pencils for blondes.

Don't be tempted to replace a brow pencil with an eyeliner pencil. Eyeliners are formulated to be soft and malleable, making them ideal for delicate eyelids. Brow pencils, on the other hand, need to be fairly hard and smudgeproof so you can create tiny, precise strokes exactly where you need them. To get the most out of an eyebrow pencil, make short, diagonal strokes following the direction of growth of the eyebrow. Concentrate on areas where the hairs are less dense, rather than just drawing across the whole brow.

For more information on creating the perfect brow, turn to page 72.

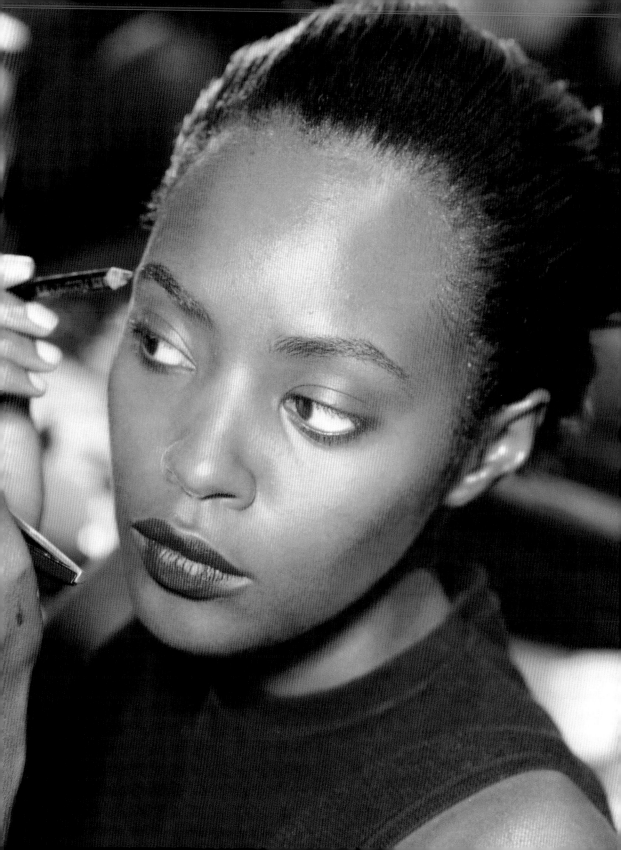

HOW TO
pluck your eyebrows

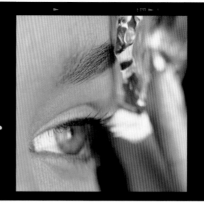

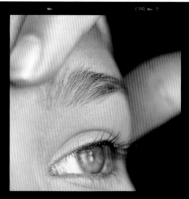

Your eyebrows frame your face, so keep them neat and tidy with regular, pain-free plucking

1 Cleanse the eyebrow area thoroughly by wiping cleanser through the brows against their direction of growth. If you are very sensitive to pain, now is the time to hold an ice cube against the area to be plucked for a few seconds.

2 Hold the skin in the brow area flat and taut between the finger and thumb of your free hand. This will help minimize discomfort and prevent the skin from being pulled with the hair when you tweeze it.

HOW TO
shade your eyebrows

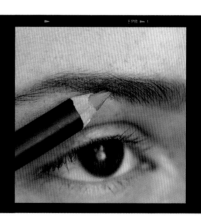

When you have the right shape, add further definition with a pencil, eyeshadow or mascara

1 The most common way to define brows is to use a pencil. Choose one that's a shade lighter than your hair colour, making sure the tip is sharpened to a point. Work along the brow using short, diagonal, upward strokes.

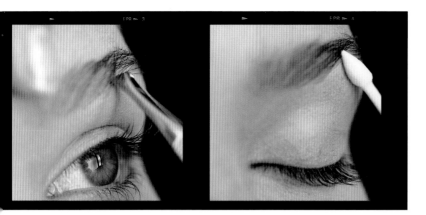

3 Grab the selected hair with clean tweezers and hold it slightly away from the brow. This will allow you to check that you want to remove that particular one before you actually take the plunge and do so.

4 Once you are happy with the shape of your tweezed brow, swab the entire area with a cotton bud soaked in alcohol-based toner or witch hazel to ensure that no bacteria penetrate the exposed follicles.

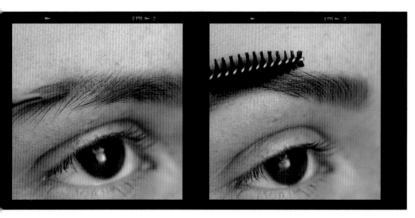

2 Eyeshadow is great for eyebrow grooming, as long as you choose a subtle shade. Brush the brow hairs downwards, then trace along the browbone with a narrow brush. Then brush the hairs back up and over the shadow.

3 If you have naturally dark brows, you can use brown waterproof mascara to add definition. Brush the hairs away from the browbone, then give them a light coat of mascara. Leave to dry for a few seconds, then gently comb them through.

brush
STROKES

A buyer's guide to make-up brushes

- Most brushes have either synthetic or natural bristles. Although modern synthetics are now very good, natural bristles are best, with sable the first choice of most make-up artists.
- Always test a brush by brushing it quickly over the back of your hand to make sure it doesn't shed too many bristles as you use it.
- Check the bristles are tightly packed. Cheaper brushes tend to have loosely packed bristles and fewer of them.

Although many make-up artists prefer to use their fingers when applying cosmetics – they are artists, after all, and have had years of experience – most agree that for the average woman, a truly professional look is more easily achieved with brushes that are specially designed for the job. Even make-up minimalists should have a few brushes in their basic kit.

There are two main reasons for this. The first is that shaped make-up brushes are the key to blending, which is the secret of really good-looking make-up. Fingertips can never create a really smooth finish. Not only do they transfer oils from your skin to your make-up, which can make it blotchy, but they also deposit oil on your blushers and shadows, sealing them and making it difficult to pick up powder the next time, even with a brush. Secondly, a brush will allow you to control the amount of powder, blusher or shadow you transfer from the pot to your skin. Do as the professionals do and, once you have loaded your brush with powder, sweep it across the back of your hand. This removes any excess and helps you assess the shade on your skin as opposed to in the pot.

So brushes are the key to better-looking make-up, but which ones are the best? Short, stubby brushes may look cute but long-handled ones are much more suitable for make-up application. This is simply because they are better balanced – the handle acts as a counterweight so the brush doesn't wobble around as you use it. A medium-thick handle should feel comfortable in your hand and still allow for precision movement, while stubby, chunky-handled brushes will be harder to control, even for face powder.

A SOUND INVESTMENT?

Spending money on a good set of brushes isn't as frivolous as it may sound. A good-quality eyeshadow will be about half the price of a decent brush, but the brush will last much longer. And anyone who has tried using the sponge-tipped applicators that come with some shadows will know that they are inflexible and impossible to control. You don't have to buy a full set of brushes at once. Treat yourself to a new one occasionally and before long you'll have all you need. Alternatively, you could go for one of the collections put together by a professional make-up artist.

Once you've taken the plunge and bought yourself some decent brushes, it's important to take care of them. Keeping them clean is obviously a good idea from a hygiene point of view, but it also helps the brushes do their job. An eyeshadow brush, for example, will retain a certain amount of powder colour every time you use it, so if it isn't cleaned, every shade you apply will end up looking muddy.

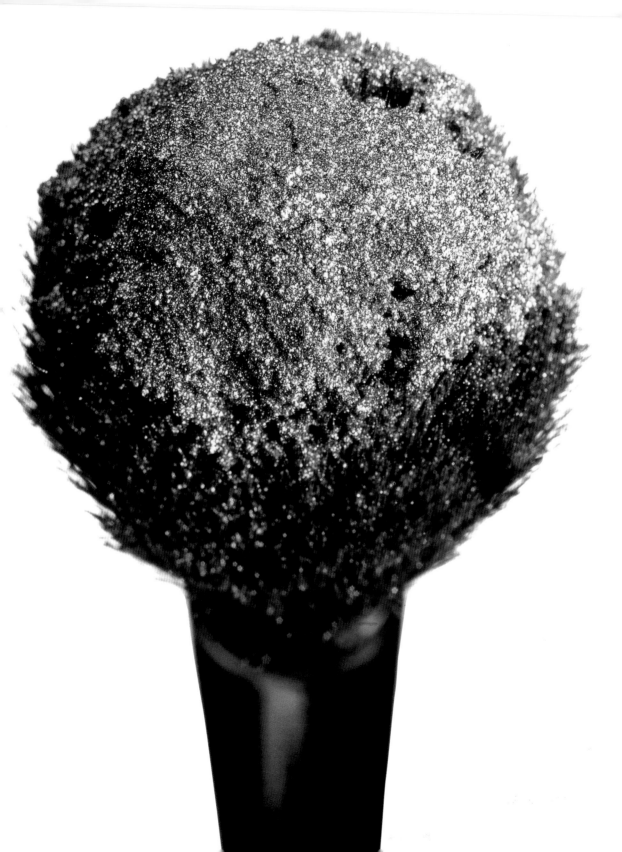

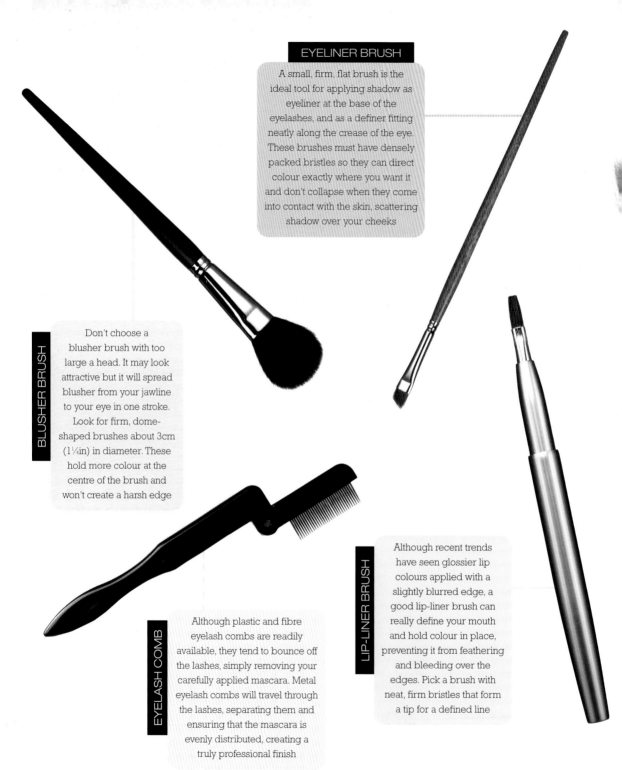

EYELINER BRUSH

A small, firm, flat brush is the ideal tool for applying shadow as eyeliner at the base of the eyelashes, and as a definer fitting neatly along the crease of the eye. These brushes must have densely packed bristles so they can direct colour exactly where you want it and don't collapse when they come into contact with the skin, scattering shadow over your cheeks

BLUSHER BRUSH

Don't choose a blusher brush with too large a head. It may look attractive but it will spread blusher from your jawline to your eye in one stroke. Look for firm, dome-shaped brushes about 3cm (1¼in) in diameter. These hold more colour at the centre of the brush and won't create a harsh edge

EYELASH COMB

Although plastic and fibre eyelash combs are readily available, they tend to bounce off the lashes, simply removing your carefully applied mascara. Metal eyelash combs will travel through the lashes, separating them and ensuring that the mascara is evenly distributed, creating a truly professional finish

LIP-LINER BRUSH

Although recent trends have seen glossier lip colours applied with a slightly blurred edge, a good lip-liner brush can really define your mouth and hold colour in place, preventing it from feathering and bleeding over the edges. Pick a brush with neat, firm bristles that form a tip for a defined line

The basic make-up kit should include five or six good-quality brushes. Whether you make eyes, lips, cheeks or brows a focal point, using the right brush will ensure the best results

EYESHADOW BRUSH

The ideal kit should contain at least one eyeshadow brush, about 1.5cm (½in) thick. A slim brush can be stroked along the delicate lid, while a slightly rounded one is best for blending

POWDER BRUSH

Powder puffs are fine for evening make-up but for daywear, a good powder brush will give a more delicate dusting. Choose a medium-sized brush rather than an absolutely enormous one, and make sure it has semi-firm bristles. If they are too floppy, they won't whisk away excess powder effectively

EYEBROW BRUSH

Eyebrow brushes need firm bristles to groom and control the short brow hairs. A soft brush will simply slide over the surface

HOW TO
conceal blemishes

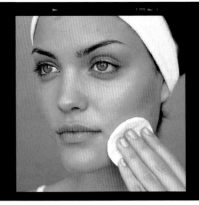

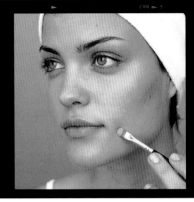

Cover up spots and blemishes with carefully applied concealer for the perfect make-up base

1 First prepare the area for concealer by cleansing and patting dry. Gently exfoliate or rub away any dry skin and ensure the area is free of oils to give the concealer the best surface to cling to.

2 Load the tip of a small, flat brush with concealer cream, depositing any excess on the back of your clean hand. Dab the concealer over the blemish itself, then clean the brush head on a tissue and use it to blend the concealer into your skin.

HOW TO
conceal shadows

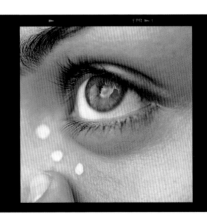

Under-eye shadows are easy to disguise – all you need is a light touch and a little expertise

1 Dot concealer from the bridge of your nose to halfway under the eye, keeping it close to the eye socket. Blend lightly, avoiding the edges of your eyes, where the concealer will sit in crows' feet.

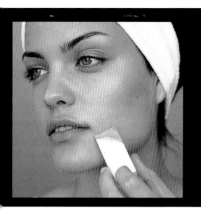

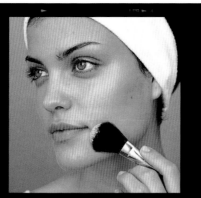

3 Using a sponge – your fingertips contain natural oils that may remove the concealer – dot your foundation over the area. If the blemish is still visible, apply another layer of concealer at this stage.

4 Finally, set your foundation with a light dusting of translucent powder. Try to resist the temptation to touch the area as you will only undo all your careful work.

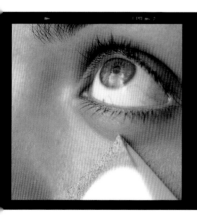

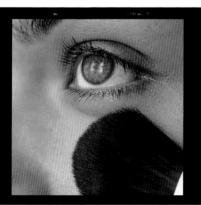

2 Sponge your foundation over the area, right up to the lower lashes. Look up into a mirror as you do so – this action will pull out any creases, which ensures better coverage.

3 Take your powder brush but, rather than dipping it into fresh powder, use the powder already clinging to the bristles to create an ultra-fine layer that will seal the concealer without leaving the area looking dry or crêpey.

HOW TO
apply
foundation

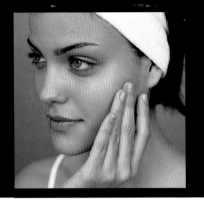

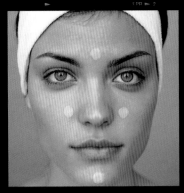

The secret of great foundation lies in its application. Get it right and you'll have a flawless finish

1 To create a smooth base for foundation, first apply a layer of moisturizer or primer all over your face and neck. Work it into the nooks and crannies, then leave for a few minutes to be fully absorbed.

2 Dot on your foundation, concentrating it in the centre of your face where most coverage is required. This will also make it easier to blend thoroughly at the edges.

HOW TO
apply
powder

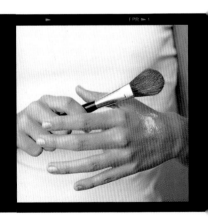

When it comes to powder, remember the golden rule – less is definitely more

1 Load your powder brush with loose powder and lightly flick it on the back of your hand a couple of times. This helps get rid of any excess before the bristles actually touch your face.

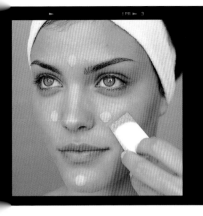

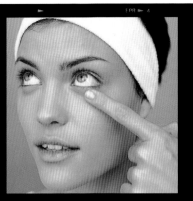

3 Using a sponge, work the foundation over the central panel of your face and out to the edges. Remember to work right around your nostrils and lightly over your ears.

4 To create a youthful, wide-awake look, use your fingertips to apply a slightly lighter foundation under your eyes. This is most effective on dark skin, but make sure the shade difference is only slight.

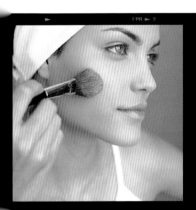

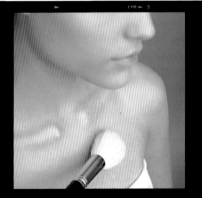

2 Begin with light movements over the central panels of your face before moving around the edges. Lightly push powder into the areas around your nostrils, then dust your eyelids and ears.

3 Highlighting powder is great for an evening look, provided it is used sparingly. So make sure your brush isn't overloaded, then stroke it over your cheekbones, shoulders, collarbone and décolletage.

finger
TIPS

Three steps to beautiful nails

- Prior to applying nail colour, sweep your nails with some nail polish remover. It helps to remove surface oils and enables the colour to adhere to the nail itself.

- To make your nails appear more slender, apply a dark varnish down the centre panel of the nail but don't take it all the way out to the edges. This creates a very effective optical illusion.

- Rather than remove all your nail polish if you make a mistake, invest in a nail corrector pen, which can be used to tidy up the edges of polished nails and get rid of any blobs of polish.

Your hands, like your face, need care and attention to look their best. And nails have become such a beauty focal point that caring for them has also become an essential part of total grooming. Treat your hands as tools of self-expression – with a simple sweep, a minimal but modern French manicure can be replaced with a dark, dramatic colour, so you can have as much fun with your nails as you dare. And why not?

Your hands are at the mercy of the environment, and they are actually a better indicator of age than a well-cared-for face. And the old cliché about wearing rubber gloves to protect them while you do the washing up is as valid as ever – hot water dries out the natural oils in your nails, making them brittle and likely to break before they grow to any length. The detergents in washing-up liquid will have the same effect, and they'll dry out your skin, too. So wear your rubber gloves, put sunscreen on your hands even when you're going to work, and treat them to nourishing creams that will protect them from wrinkles and age spots.

When applying oils or creams, be sure to work them into your nails as well as the skin of your hands. You don't have to buy expensive products to keep your hands in good condition – almond oil makes an excellent softening and nourishing treatment for both your hands and nails. Watch

your diet, too. If it is lacking in vitamins, especially oil-based ones such as E and A, you may have lacklustre, dry nails.

NATURAL NAILCARE

Never giving your nails a break from polish, however gentle, will also have a negative effect on their condition. Like skin and hair, nails need a breather, so treat them to a weekend off from time to time. You can always use a nail buffer to create chemical-free shine if you don't like the natural look.

Choose mild nailcare products when you can. Acetone-free nail polish removers, for example, are less harsh and drying to the nail itself than the stronger varieties. Toluene-free nail polishes are now also more widely available so ask for them at the beauty counters. Toluene used to be a vital ingredient in most nail polishes, but because it is fairly harsh, many companies have introduced gentler formulations, which are especially good for dry, brittle nails or irritated cuticles caused by sensitivity to polish.

Nails need filing and reshaping every seven to ten days to prevent them from breaking and fraying. Use a chunky emery board that isn't too abrasive, and never saw backwards and forwards. For really healthy-looking nails, apply a coat of polish with a slight hint of pink, which will counter their natural, yellowy undertones. Turn to page 84 for more nailcare tips.

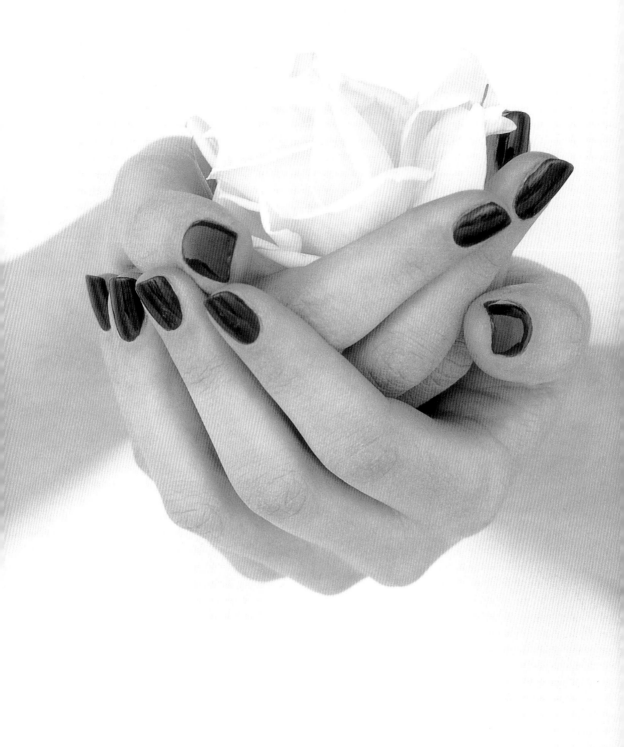

HOW TO
manicure nails

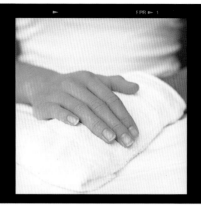

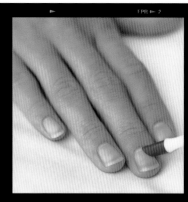

For strong, healthy nails that look neat and groomed, treat yourself to a regular manicure

1 Coat freshly washed hands in a generous layer of almond oil or your regular hand lotion. Then wrap each hand in a warm towel and relax for 15 minutes. To enhance the effect, you can cover your hands in clingfilm before wrapping them in towels.

2 Unwrap your hands and gently push back the cuticles, which will have been softened by the oils. Use a rubber hoof or cuticle stone rather than cuticle clippers, which can nick the skin and leave it open to infection.

HOW TO
apply French polish

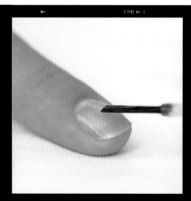

This is a real modern classic, an elegant finish that can be created with just a few simple strokes

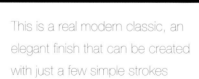

1 First file your nails – a French manicure looks best on a fairly square-tipped nail, so don't create too much of a point at the centre. Once your nails are the desired shape, apply a base coat.

masterclass

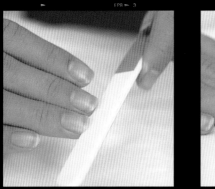

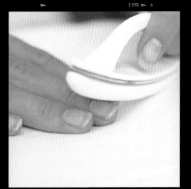

3 Next, file your nails. Keep the file moving in clean, one-directional sweeps across your nails rather than using sawing movements. Avoid metal files, which can drag if not handled professionally. Instead, use a smooth, fine emery board that will slide easily.

4 If you want a shiny finish but don't have time to paint your nails, simply buff them with a nail buff, which will create a natural, glossy look.

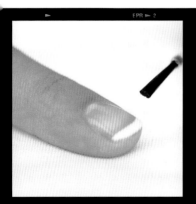

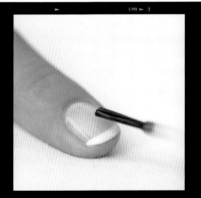

2 The trickiest part of a French manicure is creating the whitened tip. Lay the hand to be painted on a flat surface in front of you and keep the ball of your painting hand steady by resting it on the same surface. Then just drag the brush tip straight across the nail.

3 Finally, apply a coat of translucent shell-pink polish to seal the whitened tip and complete the effect. For a more modern version of the French manicure, apply a transparent beige top coat.

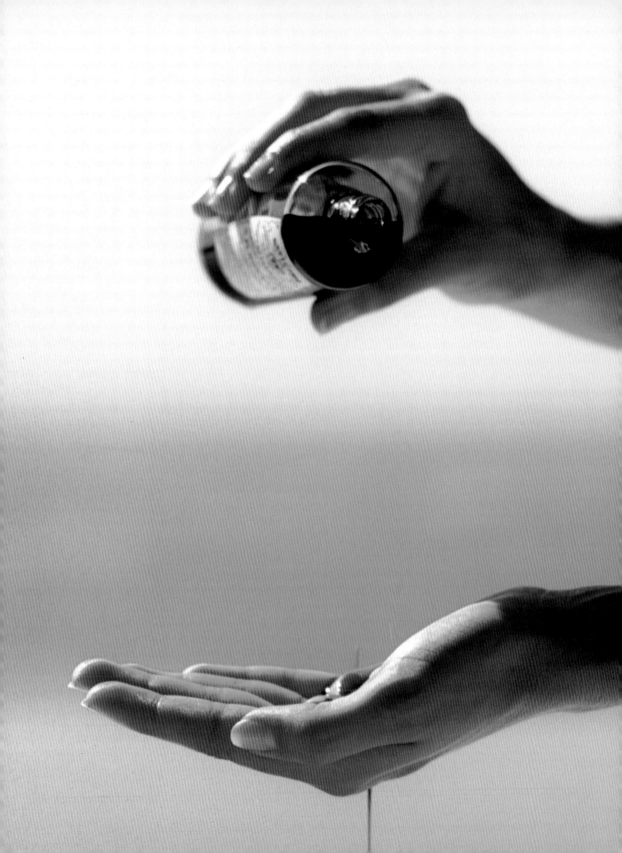

faking
IT

The dangers the sun poses to our health are well-known. At best it damages our skin and accelerates the ageing process; at worst it can cause skin cancer. Yet we still associate sun-kissed skin with health, vitality and sensuality. A golden tan makes us feel better and look better, or so we believe. It makes our eyes look brighter, our teeth whiter and our complexions less blotchy. It even seems to disguise the dreaded cellulite on our thighs. But the truth is that fake-tanning technology has been refined to such a degree that the tan from a tube now looks as good as the real thing, and has all the psychological advantages with none of the hazardous side effects.

WHAT IS FAKE TAN?

Dihydroxyacetone or DHA is the key ingredient in most fake-tanning products. A natural sugar derived from grapes, it reacts with proteins in the skin's surface layer to produce a colour change. The greater the quantity of DHA in a product, the greater the colour change. But the chemical cannot penetrate the skin's lower layers so it is unlikely to cause an allergic reaction, even in sensitive skin.

The time it takes for a fake tan to develop on the skin varies from one product to another, but some modern formulas take as little as 20 minutes to create a golden glow that lasts for anything from three days to a week. Look for brands that offer varying intensities of tan so you can start off with the lightest shade. See how it looks on your skin, then build it up gradually if you want a deeper tan. That way you won't look as if you've been on a two-week holiday overnight.

If you have oily skin, make the most of designated products and invest in one for an oily complexion and another for a less oily body. This will ensure better results than one unsuitable compromise.

HOW TO APPLY IT

Follow the simple steps outlined below for swift, effective fake tanning.

Face Cleanse your skin thoroughly, making sure you remove all residue cleanser. If you want to use a moisturizer first, do so only sparingly and give it plenty of time to sink into the skin. Although many of us apply tanning lotions before we go to bed, in the hope that we'll wake up a healthy shade of gold, some experts recommend applying face fakes in the morning. This gives them a chance to be absorbed evenly without the interference of a pillow, which may rub the lotion off.

Body Have a good exfoliating scrubdown before applying any fake-tanning products, paying particular attention to areas that are prone to dry skin, such as the ankles,

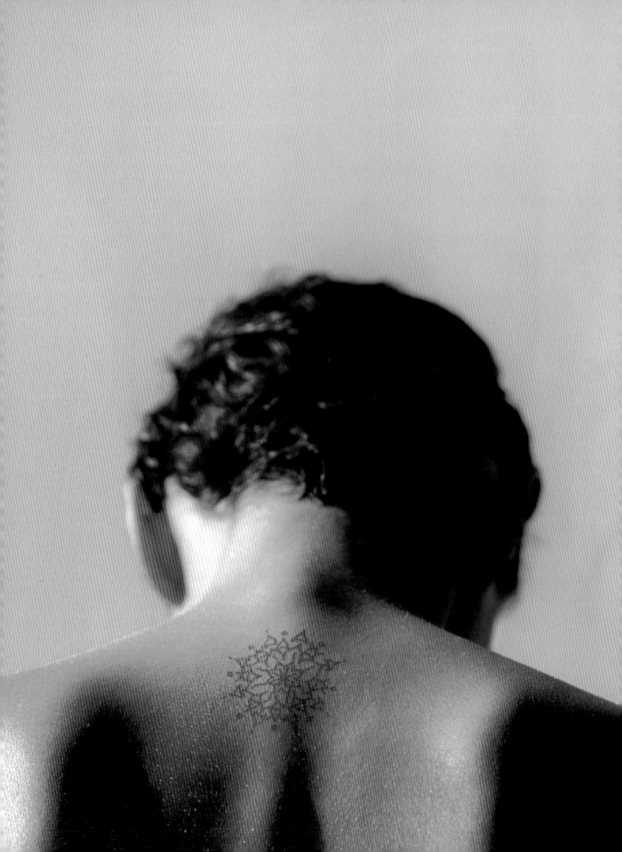

knees and elbows. Shaving your legs the day before applying fake tan also helps avoid tan blotches. If you have dry skin, apply a thin layer of moisturizer but allow it time to sink in completely before applying your fake tan.

Hands It's important to wash your hands thoroughly after applying a fake tan to avoid dark, tanned palms. Equally, though, it's worth remembering to reapply the lotion to the backs of your hands to avoid strangely pale extremities. The easiest way to do this is to pull the backs of your cleaned hands across your freshly coated legs, which will lightly recover them.

Feet For a realistic tan around your feet, concentrate the colour on the surface of the foot only, and then take a cotton-wool ball dotted with moisturizer and wipe it gently round the edge of the foot to fade the colour down in a natural-looking way.

Finally, remember that while fake tans may be the safest route to golden skin, they don't all provide protection from the sun's rays. So if the fake tan you buy doesn't have a good SPF, make sure you use a separate sunscreen on top.

TEMPORARY MEASURES

The really faint-hearted can achieve an even more temporary tan with tinted gels and creams that work instantly but can be washed off. The colour is visible as you apply it so there's no nail-biting waiting and, if you don't like the results, you can get rid of them straight away. Again, start cautiously, applying a little product to a large area. Build it up by layering more colour over the area as desired. Tinted gels work best on well-moisturized skin as dry skin will create a patchy finish. For the same reason, be sure to lightly buff away any areas of flaky skin before you start. For a totally realistic effect on the face, build intensity on the bony areas – across the cheekbones, the forehead and over the nose. Because of their prominence, these areas naturally catch the sun more easily.

Tinted moisturizers are ingenious little beauty products and no self-respecting summer make-up kit should be without one. Due to their popularity in the summer months, these moisturizers often contain SPFs, but still check the labels thoroughly.

For a youthful halo effect, smooth a little tinted gel at the top of your forehead, blending it into the hairline. Then take some tinted moisturizer on your fingertips and apply it from the bridge of your nose out over your cheeks to the sides of your face. This creates a sunkissed look that will also emphasize your bone structure.

Blend the tinted moisturizer gently up to the eye, but don't apply it directly over this area as it often looks unrealistic. If you want slightly heavier coverage, apply the tinted moisturizer with a sponge – this will create more intense colour.

TIP If you need a quick fix because you have overdone a tinted moisturizer or developing fake tan, dilute the effect by quickly rubbing your regular moisturizer over the entire area.

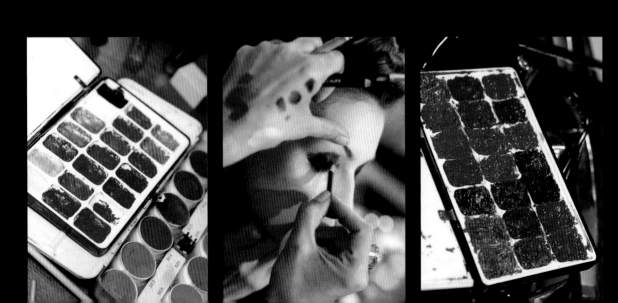

colour

NATURAL
neutrals

Whether you have a passion for make-up or not, you probably have a basic set of shadows and lip colours that you know and love. These colours give you the freedom to experiment and be creative, to match your make-up to your mood and put the finishing touches to your perfectly applied base.

The chances are, however, that most of your favourite shades are neutral tones. Neutral shades are great basics – they're reliable and user-friendly, and they're unlikely to go out of date and end up buried at the bottom of your make-up drawer. Wild, new colours may appear each year on the catwalks, but our tried-and-tested neutrals are the ones we usually turn to on a daily basis.

Neutrals should be viewed as enhancers, so work with your natural skin and hair colouring when choosing shades for yourself. Chocolate browns, for example, won't look neutral on a fair-haired, fair-skinned woman, while pastel pinks will be equally unsuitable for a darker complexion (turn to page 94 for a more detailed shade guide for your skin tone). Next, take a close look at the colour of your eyes and, if you have a drawer full of neutral eyeshadows, try to whittle them down. Apply them one at a time next to your eye to see which looks best. Badly chosen neutrals can actually look flat and deaden your natural colours, rather than emphasizing them, so it's important to identify those that work for you.

Although neutrals are background colours, they don't have to be matt. In fact, beige-coloured creams and ivories can look quite chalky when they're totally matt but are brought to life by subtle sheen. For the same reason, taupes and mushrooms may work better in cream rather than powder formulations. To assess a colour's sheen, apply it to the back of your hand and move it around under a direct light. This quickly shows whether it is either too matt or too sparkly.

The same principles apply to lipsticks. Glosses used to be seen as natural, but many now contain highly iridescent particles, which makes them more suitable for dramatic evening looks. Again, consider your natural lip colour when choosing neutral shades for lips. Try to stick to the same tone, whether it's a slightly burnished red or a flesh pink, but increase the intensity of colour when you want to accentuate the effect.

Neutral shades really come into their own when your skin looks a little tired and wan. When vibrant colour would be too extreme, a subtle rosy blush will give your face a lift. Lip sheens and satins also work wonders on days like these, providing a touch of much-needed radiance.

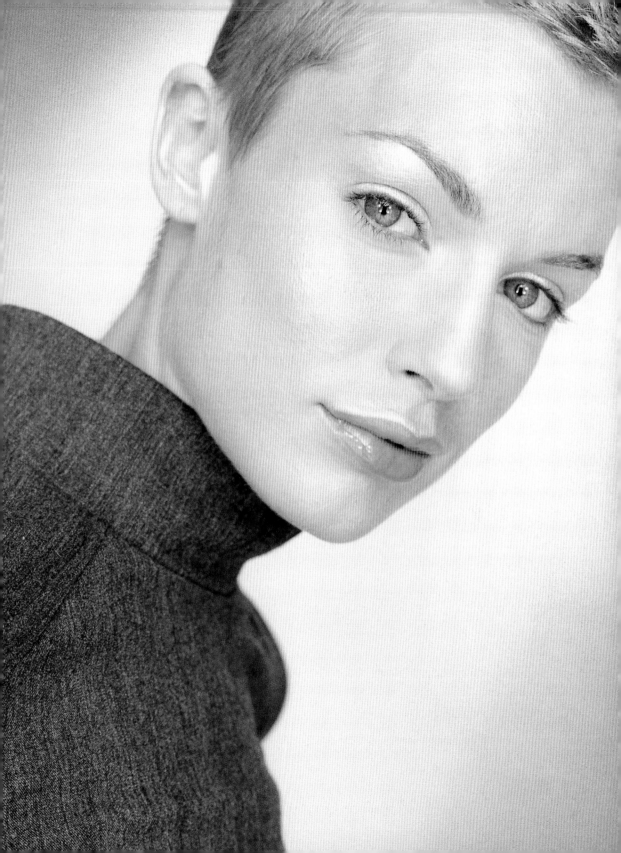

THE NEUTRAL PALETTE

Neutrals may be subtle, but they can still transform eyes, cheeks, lips and nails. The secret is to choose those that will flatter your colouring as well as your individual features.

EYESHADOW   POWDER BLUSHER

PALE SKIN, RED HAIR

Really pale skins benefit from neutral shades that are softly tinted with apricot, or subtle rose pinks. These avoid the wan look of true beiges

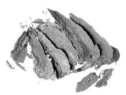
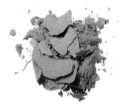

FAIR SKIN, FAIR HAIR

These complexions can look great with neutral make-up shades but, to avoid looking washed-out, make sure you use more than one shade or tone throughout

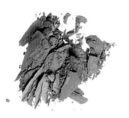
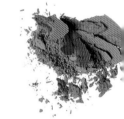

OLIVE SKIN, DARK HAIR

Olive skins require a slight contrast in colour, so choose shades that are slightly darker than your skin tone to create a neutral look

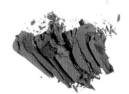
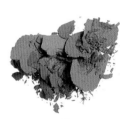

DARK SKIN, BLACK HAIR

Dark skins look best if they are highlighted with slightly shimmery neutrals and accented with dark, plummy shades

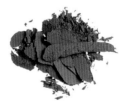

DULL SKIN, GREY HAIR

Peachy, apricot shades will add a warmer, more youthful glow to mature skins, while rosy pinks are best avoided as they can look greying

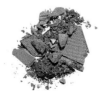
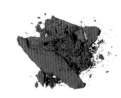

LIPSTICK   LIP PENCIL   NAIL POLISH

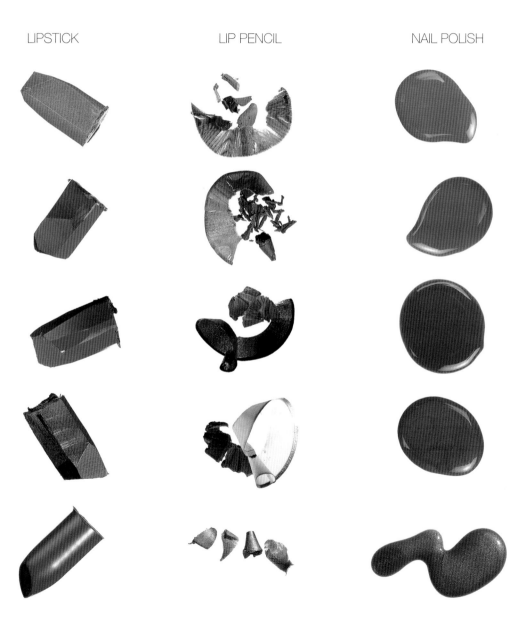

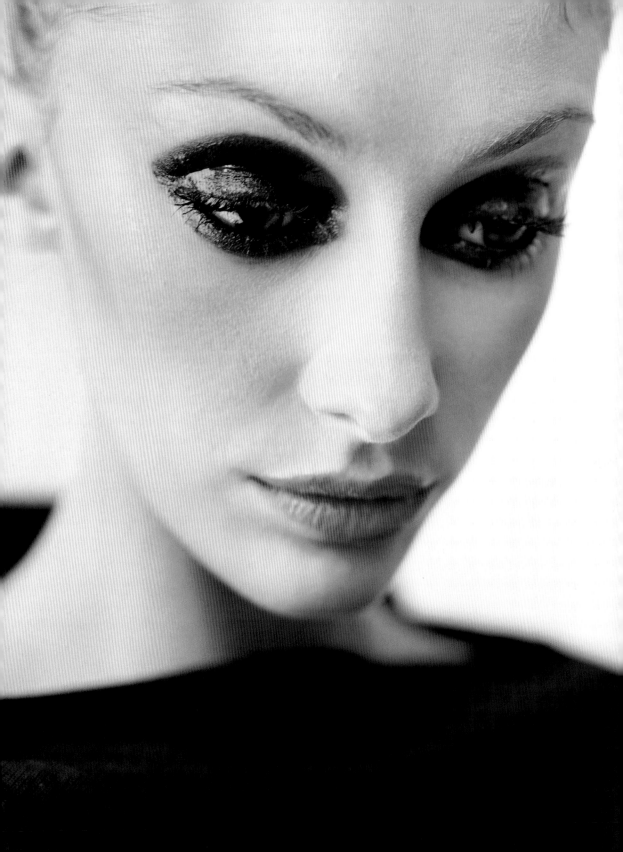

GLORIOUS
colour

A fresh, new make-up colour can transform your appearance in an instant, and it's a much cheaper way of keeping up with the season's latest looks than a new outfit. And the best thing about make-up is that it isn't permanent. You can have some fun experimenting and, if you don't like the results, you just remove them. Start at the cosmetics counters – trying out lip colours you've never dreamt of wearing, for example, can be both enjoyable and surprising.

But before you take the plunge and buy, remember that the secret of successful colour is to keep it simple. Don't overload your face with an array of different shades. Instead, focus on one element and make it as bold and vibrant as you dare. Emphasize either your eyes or lips but not both, and if the colours you choose are really bright, just add little dashes of them. Striking turquoise and purply-red shadows look wonderful applied in tiny dots or fine lines above the eyelashes, but not so good spread over the entire eyelid. On the other hand, iridescent navy blues and satiny plums work well slicked over the whole lid, as long as they are blended at the edges (see page 98 for more tips on texture and the way it affects make-up colours).

Precision application is vital with strong colours. A bright red lipstick, for instance, will never look good if it is messily applied. The intensity of the colour means it must be framed with a neat pencil line and carefully filled in with a lip brush (turn to page 114 for more details). Alternatively, why not invest in a chunky lipstick pencil that will do both jobs at the same time?

Take your complexion into account, too. Youthful skins can get away with brilliantly bright lips and just a sheeny, nearly natural finish, while older skins look better when colour is applied to a perfectly prepped base of foundation followed by a light dusting of powder.

Look at magazines for colour inspiration. Trying new things is half the fun, and will help create dynamic new looks that work for you as long as you bear a few ground rules in mind. Colourful mascaras, for instance, look best worn alone, rather than to finish an already colourful eye make-up. And they only really work on youthful complexions. Bright, intense blushers, on the other hand, are best avoided altogether as blusher is meant to be subtle. And don't go for really bright orange for cheeks, eyes or lips – it's an unnatural shade posing as a natural one, and is too harsh for most skin tones. Finally, stick to the shades you know on important days. Interviews, weddings and first dates are not the right times to experiment with colourful make-up.

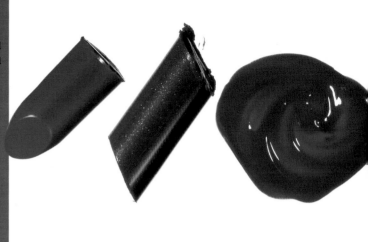

If you want a lip colour to match its tester exactly, pick a solid, matt formulation or a cream in a tube. Glossy metallics produce less concentrated colour and can be applied in a fine layer or built up gradually for greater intensity. Sheer gloss creates a stunning finish, despite its lack of colour, while coloured glosses combine the best of both worlds – vibrancy and shine. Their light-refracting qualities mean they look most dramatic at night

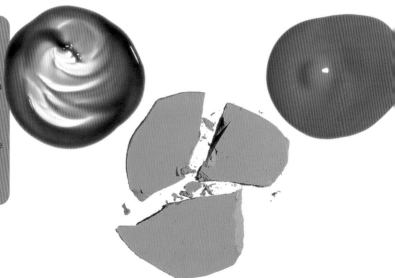

Blusher has infinite variations in texture, from barely-there to opaque. Sheer cheek gels can be blended over nude skin – their water-based formulation gives them great spread and a transparent finish, even when the colours look strong in the pot. Powder blushers are great for daywear as they create a subtle but professional finish, while cream blushers produce a wonderful, warm glow for evenings

The texture of any make-up shade will influence the way it looks on your skin, so take time to compare the different finishes, from matt powders to sheer or tinted glosses, iridescent creams to translucent colour washes

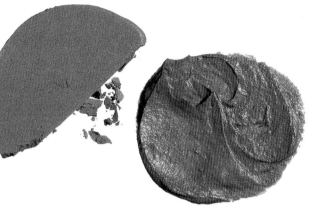

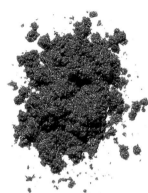

EYES

Eyes get the biggest hit of colour from loose-powder formulations, which are very pigment-rich. Most pressed shadows are now creamy enough to be blended easily, even when they are powder, so a colour that looks very intense in the compact may not appear so on the skin. Cream shadows need only be dotted on to the eyelid as they spread a long way, which also makes them easy to blend. Sparkly shades, which can be overpowering for daywear, will look great worn at night

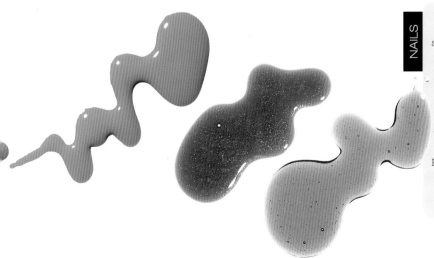

NAILS

The newest nail polishes are translucent washes, which look strong in the pot but much less so on your nails. Their seethrough nature gives them a very watery depth, and they won't contrast harshly with your skin. Sparkly colours should be kept for evenings as they can look garish during the day, whereas matt polishes, another recent arrival at the beauty counters, give a serious finish to nails and are ideal for a day in the office

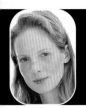

PALE, FRECKLED SKIN, RED HAIR

see page 21

Pale, freckled skin like Arabella's has some inherent difficulties when it comes to make-up. Freckles look best under **sheer foundation**, and it's much more sensible to let them show rather than to try to blank them out with heavy base products. As these skins are rarely oily, you can **forget powder** unless you need a light dusting in the T-zone. Eyebrow pencils and shading sticks can be hard to match to a redhead's subtle complexion, but a blonde or beige-toned pencil will probably look more natural than a brown one.

There are lots of rules about which colours go best with red hair, with the standard advice being to go for subtle greens and blues on the eyes, and to opt for red-tinted lip colours. In fact, your skin tone shouldn't stop you trying anything. Muted mushroom, taupe and lilac shades, for example, work incredibly well on the eyes for a **daytime barely-there look**. Some freckled skins look wonderful with a hint of rosy-pink blusher, while others cry out for berry-stained lips.

avoid

inky-black mascara, unless your brows are well-defined

using heavy base products to hide your freckles

look for

sheer tints for lips – either stains or glosses

pale beige-toned eyebrow pencils

gel blushers, which allow freckles to show through

PICKING THE RIGHT FOUNDATION

A semi-transparent foundation in a very lightweight formulation will create the most natural effect on a pale complexion, but make sure the one you choose also provides good levels of sun protection. Not only will this help shield sensitive skin from the elements during the cooler months of the year, but it also means you won't need a separate sunscreen – and yet another chemical layer – on your skin in the summer.

Finding the right shade of foundation can be a nightmare for women with skin like Arabella's, as freckles are obviously darker than the rest of the face. The best idea is to choose one that matches your dominant shade, which in most cases is the paler one. This also makes it easier to blend the foundation in the neck area, where most people have fewer freckles.

TIP Giving skin a rest from make-up from time to time is always a good idea, but it is especially beneficial for this type of skin, which tends to be sensitive

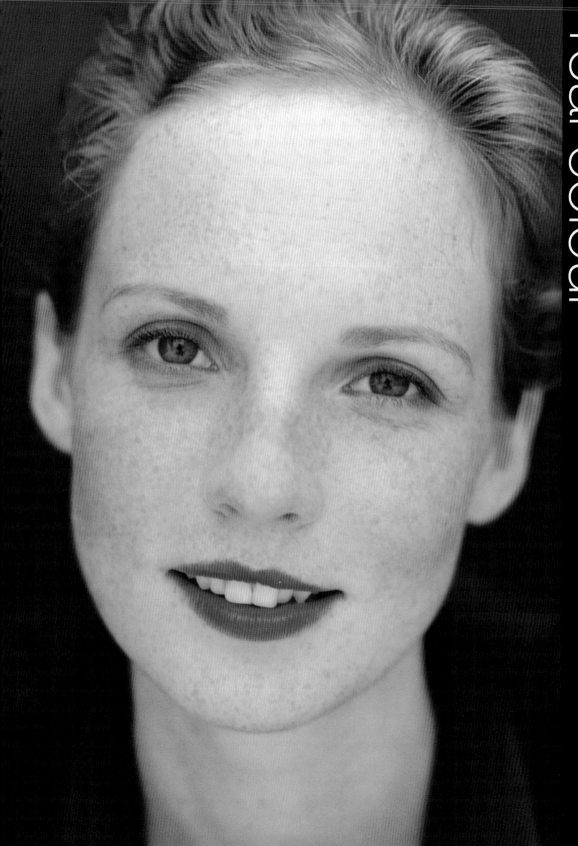

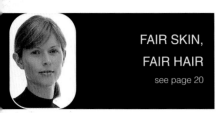

FAIR SKIN, FAIR HAIR
see page 20

The main difficulty with fair skin like Jo's is working out whether it has **warm or cool undertones**. A warm, fair skin will look washed-out if you apply cool shades, such as pastel pinks, muted lilacs and pale mushroom tones. On the other hand, warm colours, such as mellow golden browns, will lift it and give it a gentle glow. And for cool-toned skins the reverse is true.

Avoid pale blue eyeshadow, whatever your skin tone. It will detract from your eyes rather than enhancing them – even if they are blue – and tends to look dated. **Contrasting neutral shades** are a much better bet, and will really bring out your eye colour. Terracotta or orange-toned blushers are also too overpowering for pale skin so steer clear of them. Instead, try a warm apricot or cool rosy pink to bring **colour to your cheeks**. And for your lips, opt for either transparent, warm browny-pinks or cool lilac-pinks, which will add subtle drama without going overboard.

avoid

matt shades – they'll look dull against your skin

orange-toned blushers, which are too overpowering

look for

shimmering neutral shades to emphasize your eyes

transparent lip colours, which won't look too heavy

dark brown mascaras for daywear

CREATING INSTANT DRAMA

Rather than overwhelming your eyes with dark, smoky looks, try this shimmery look for evenings. Applying the cool versus warm tone principle, take either a silver or gold cream shadow. Apply it over your eyelid and blend well up to the browbone, but use it sparingly – a little of either of these colours will go a long way. Don't add any colour to the browbone itself, but dot with a tiny amount of petroleum jelly for a slick finish. Then use a creamy highlighter over your cheekbones, moving in a crescent around the outer areas of your eyes. Warm your cheeks with a cream blusher and define lips with a cool, sheer raspberry stain or a rich, red, frosted cream lipstick applied with a lip brush. Finally, add definition to your brows with a mid-brown eyeshadow applied along the browline – this is a softer alternative to pencil.

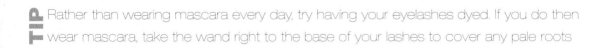

TIP Rather than wearing mascara every day, try having your eyelashes dyed. If you do then wear mascara, take the wand right to the base of your lashes to cover any pale roots

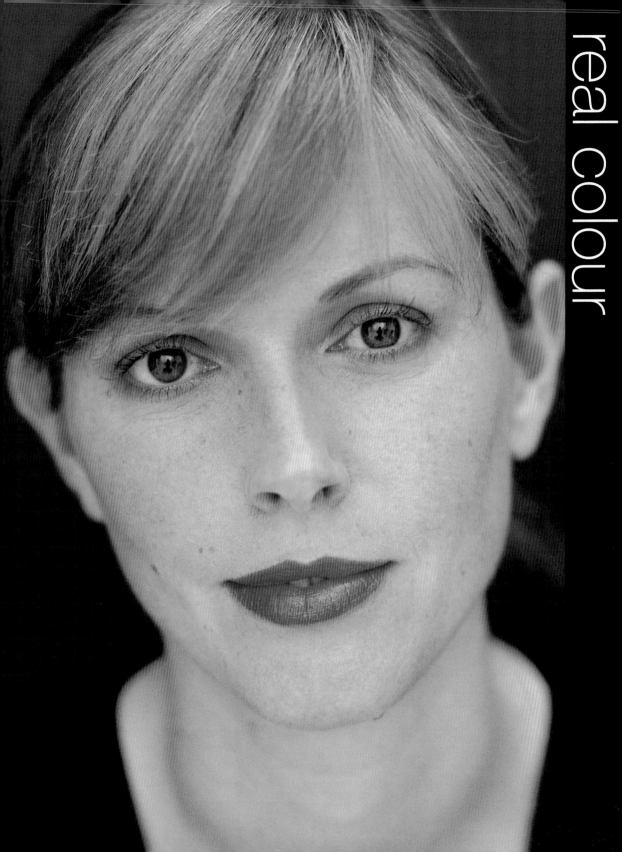

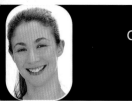

OLIVE SKIN, DARK HAIR
see page 21

The last thing skin such as Susanna's needs is oil-rich make-up. Instead, use a primer to create a **shine-free, non-slip base** and follow with a mattifying foundation. These usually contain starches that will mop up any oils the skin produces. **Warm, yellow-toned foundation** will complement olive skin, whereas pink-toned bases will appear to float on its surface. Compare the two at a cosmetic counter and you'll see what a difference the right shade makes. **Loose powder is another essential** for oily skin. Modern formulations are so fine they won't clog your skin, but don't overdo it – a fine dusting looks much more beautiful than a thick layer.

Olive skins look good with a whole range of colours. Opt for dark eyeliner, bold lipstick and dramatic Latin shades, or go for shimmering pastels on your eyes. Pale pink, frosted lip colours are probably the only thing that won't suit you. Try **sheer lip shades** instead – they'll divert attention from any shine on your skin.

avoid

orange-toned blushers, which will make the skin look sallow

pink-toned base products and pale pink lip colours

look for

absorbent face papers to soak up excess oils

rich berry shades for lips

soft eyeliner pencils for above and beneath the lashes

A TOUCH OF EVENING GLAMOUR

For a wonderful evening look, try a pearlized eyeshadow or cream in jade or pale turquoise. Keep the colour pure and just use it on the upper lid, blending into a creamy highlighter on the browbone. Create a dramatic browline with a pencil and then define the eyes with lashings of mascara. Finish with a slick of moisturizing lipstick in a muted browny beige.

Alternatively, intensify your natural, dark colouring by creating smouldering eyes. Blend darker to lighter shadows from the lashes up to the browbone, before using liquid eyeliner very close to the upper lashes along the length of the lid. Apply a mid-toned eyeshadow using an eyeliner brush beneath the lower lashes. Finish with jet-black mascara.

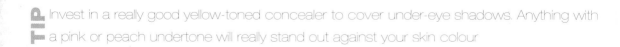

TIP Invest in a really good yellow-toned concealer to cover under-eye shadows. Anything with a pink or peach undertone will really stand out against your skin colour

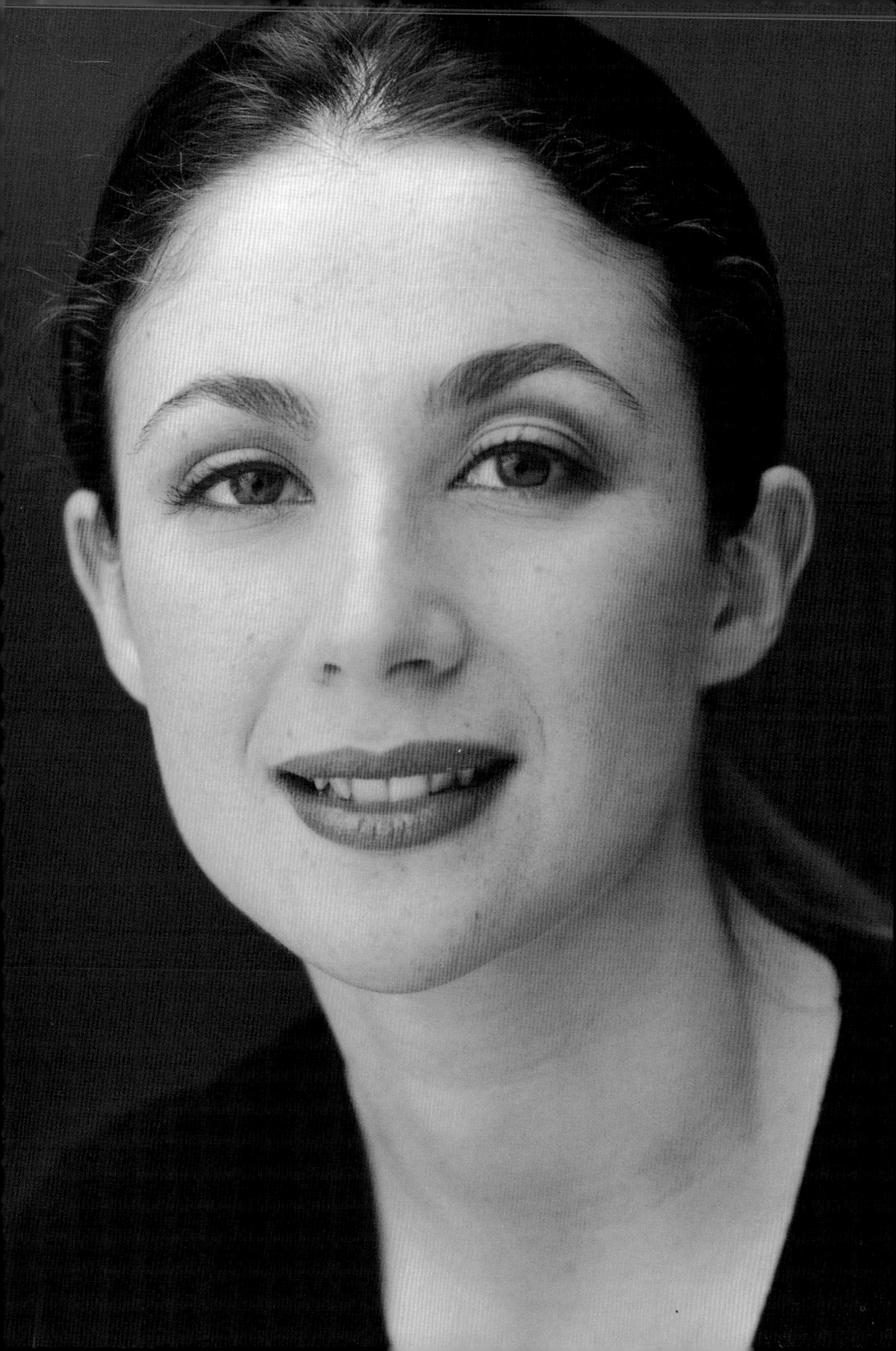

real colour

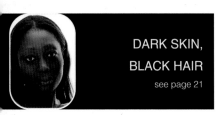

DARK SKIN, BLACK HAIR

see page 21

Few make-up ranges are specifically designed for dark skins such as Sandra's, but their numbers are growing. This is good news because while paler skins absorb the **chalky powder particles** that underlie all make-up colours, these same substances show up on darker skins, diluting the colour of the shadow and creating an ashy look. So while **gels, sheers and transparent** eye, cheek and lip colours work on all skins, shadow and powder colours should be chosen from ranges devised for darker skins. They will contain much higher pigment levels, which ensure the colours stay true on the skin.

Dark skins can look wonderful with **dramatic make-up shades**, such as navy and rich purple, both of which will make your eyes look whiter. Choose colours with a **slight iridescence**, which will flatter rather than flatten your skin tone. And to give greater symmetry to the mouth, try applying your favourite lip colour and then adding a tiny bit of concealer over the top of the upper lip.

avoid

matt lip colours, which will make the mouth look very flat

very oily foundations, which will emphasize shiny skin

look for

plummy, slightly pearlized blushers

sheer, berry lip shades for a soft, sumptuous mouth

iridescent eyeshadow colours for real drama

SCULPT AND SHIMMER

For a supermodel-inspired sculpted look, apply a shade of foundation that's slightly paler than normal in the under-eye area, blending it carefully towards the cheekbones. Then use either a darker shade or a bronzing stick to create depth under the cheekbones, and finish with your regular foundation. This technique has the double advantage of making your cheekbones stand out a mile as well as drawing attention to the eye area.

Darker skins can also afford to mix and match their foundation and powder colours. By applying a base colour that matches the skin's natural tone exactly, and then sweeping a slightly lighter layer of powder over it, you can create a wonderfully luminous texture on the skin. For an evening look, you can try this using a slightly shimmery powder.

 For really dramatic evening eyes, use a black or aubergine liquid liner to accent the eye and create a dense, slick finish. Pencils won't be nearly as visible

real colour

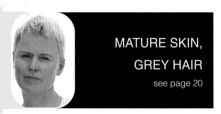

MATURE SKIN, GREY HAIR

see page 20

Older women like Lynne tend to be more preoccupied with skincare than make-up. And while a great skincare routine can transform dull, mature skin, make-up, too, can create a more **modern youthful** appearance. If this applies to you, it is probably time for reassessment. Are you clinging to old habits? Do you choose colour that could be updated either in texture or shade?

Start with one of the new **light-reflective foundations** which will really lift your skin. Grey hair can subtly change the skin undertones, making them appear slightly cool, so counteract this with apricot- and peach-coloured blushers, and yellowy pink-toned powder. Don't think you can't wear dramatic make-up, though. Deep reds can look wonderful with pale skin and grey hair. Equally, muted rose shades will **enhance the lips** while diverting attention to the eyes. Eyes themselves can look striking. Experiment with smoky colours above and below the eye, always remembering to blend well.

avoid

matt formulations, which emphasize

dull skin

pink-toned powders, which can

be ageing

look for

light-reflecting pigments in foundations and powders

golden or peach-toned loose powders

creamy, moisturizing lipstick formulations

PRECISION APPLICATION

To apply make-up to older eyes, open the eye area by gently holding the eyebrow up. This allows you to apply shadow all over the lid, rather than just the part that's visible. Before you start, moisturize thoroughly and apply foundation using a dense sponge chip. This will help distribute it over the entire eye area and will also prevent colour from sitting in crows' feet. To boost dwindling eyelashes and emphasize the eye, use an eyelash curler first. This will intensify the effect of mascara and help open up the eye itself. Use a crisp, black mascara rather than a brown one to enhance the eye whites.

Lip liner is absolutely essential for mature skin. This is because it creates a waxy barrier that holds lip colour in place and prevents it from feathering and bleeding over the edges. For a step-by-step guide to creating the perfect lip shape, turn to page 114.

TIP Apply slightly less foundation around the far edges of the eye, where it may draw attention to fine lines and wrinkles rather than concealing them

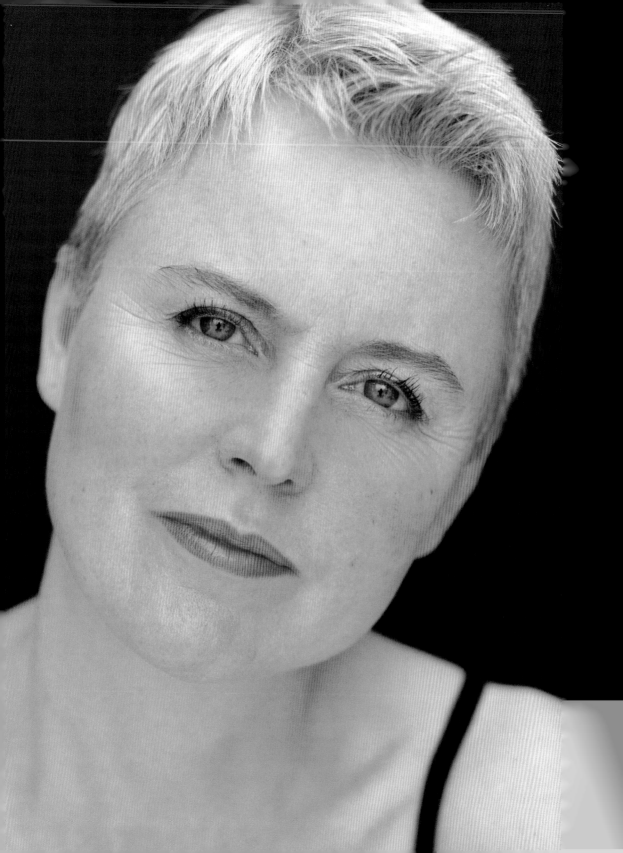

HOW TO
enhance
your eyes

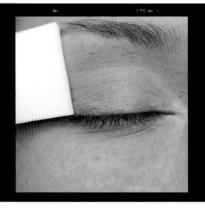

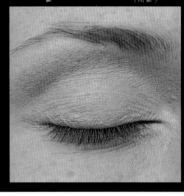

For a subtle, barely-there look, go for natural shades on your eyes and a softly shaped brow

1 If you are wearing foundation, pat or sponge a little over your eyelids. Otherwise, use a little primer to prepare the area for make-up.

2 Apply a pale, neutral colour over the entire lid, blending up to the browbone. For a modern finish, opt for a neutral shadow with a slight sheen.

HOW TO
define your
eyes

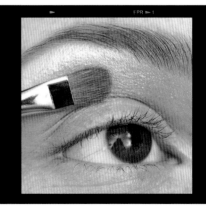

This quick and easy way of accentuating your eyes is perfect for daytime glamour

1 To create this very slick look, lightly cover your eyelids with your usual foundation, then apply a pale, lightly frosted shadow over the browbone.

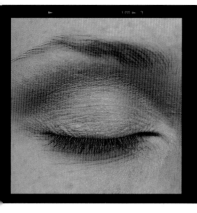

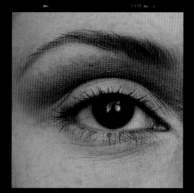

3 Take a slightly darker neutral shade and apply it along the crease or hollow of the lid, blending it carefully to avoid any hard edges.

4 You can brush a little of the same shadow through your brows to create a uniform look. Finish with a single coat of mascara, combed through to remove any excess.

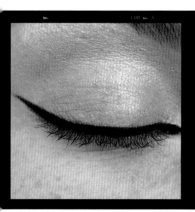

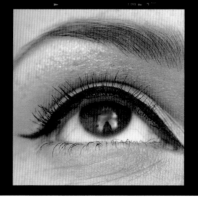

2 Trace a fine line along your upper lashes using a liquid eyeliner or, for a softer look, an eyeliner brush and dark shadow. Flick the line upwards slightly at the edge.

3 Curl your eyelashes, then apply a single coat of mascara. Finally, define your brows with an eyebrow pencil.

HOW TO
dramatize
your eyes

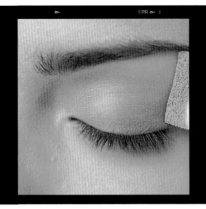

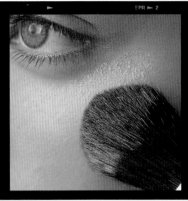

Evening is the time to get glowing, with eyes that smoulder and make-up that really shines

1 Prepare the whole eye area for make-up by applying a layer of foundation with a small sponge to work it well into the corners. Don't powder the upper lid – foundation creates a better base for colour.

2 Sweep some translucent loose powder across the top of your cheekbones, just under your eyes. This will catch any falling particles of eyeshadow, which can then be easily whisked away.

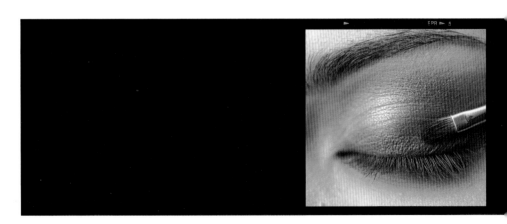

5 Taking a darker eyeshadow in a similar colour, trace along the upper lid, again working as close to the lashes as you can get. Blend it lightly into the paler shade.

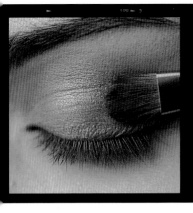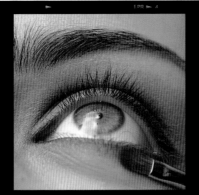

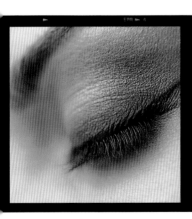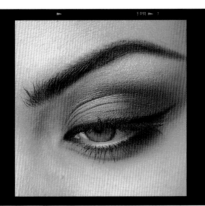

3 Apply a mid-tone shadow over the entire eyelid, taking it from the lashes up to the eye hollow. Mid-greys or plums work well for this look. Clean the brush tip and blend the colour at the edge of the eye hollow to soften any hard edges.

4 Take a small eyeshadow brush and, looking up into a mirror, apply the same shade along the lower lid, underneath the lashes but as close as you can get to them. Clean the brush tip on a tissue before blending the outer edges of this line.

6 To accentuate your eyes, trace along the upper lid next to the lashes with a dark liquid eyeliner. Work from the centre of the eye out to the far edges, flicking the line up slightly at the corner to create a feline look.

7 Finally, brush a highlighter shade across the browbone to dramatize the eye area. Define brows with pencil or shadow, then apply two light coats of mascara to the upper and lower lashes, combing through after each application.

HOW TO
emphasize your lips

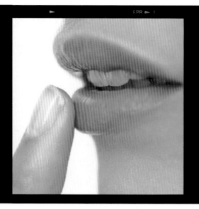

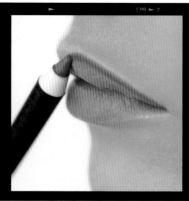

Bold lips are a great way of making a statement, but only if they are properly defined

Using the right tools helps create the most flattering lip shape as well as giving longer-lasting results. First prime your lips with a good lip cream, but avoid waxy salves. Wait for a couple of minutes for the cream to be absorbed.

Choose a lip pencil that matches your lipstick. You shouldn't be able to see the pencil line at all once the lipstick is applied – it simply creates a defined edge. Start in the centre of your upper lip and work out to the corners. For the bottom lip, work from the corners into the centre.

HOW TO
create high-shine lips

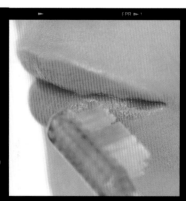

Smooth, scrubbed lips and a soft, slightly blurred outline are crucial for a really glossy finish

It is essential that your lips are fully prepped for this look, so either rub them lightly with a little face scrub or apply some lip salve and then brush them with a soft toothbrush to remove any dead or dry skin cells.

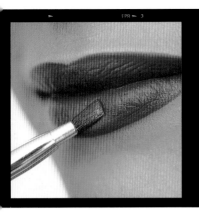

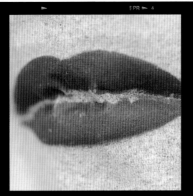

3 Fill the whole area, right up to the lip line, with lipstick. Applying it with a lip brush really helps you get into the corners of your mouth and work the colour in well.

4 Finally, blot your lips with a single layer of tissue to help fix the colour in place. There's no need to apply powder, but you may want to add another layer of colour or a slick of gloss for a richer effect.

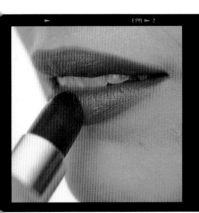

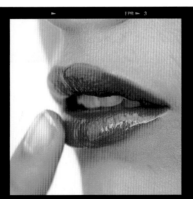

2 To give extra depth to a glossy look, apply a light coat of your regular lip colour. You can apply it straight from the tube as gloss looks better with blurred edges. There's certainly no need to use lip liner.

3 Apply the gloss straight from the pot with your fingertips. Remember that high shine will make your lips the focal point of your face, so don't overdo it.

OFFICE TO
evening

When you've been stuck in meetings or hunched over a word processor all day, it can be hard to find the time and energy to get ready for an evening out. But don't despair. A few simple tricks can restore your existing make-up in seconds, and looking good is a sure way to boost flagging energy levels. Lightness of hand is the key to a refreshed evening look, so try not to pile on too much make-up.

1 Instead of removing your entire base, sprinkle a cotton-wool pad with floral water and sweep it over your skin. This will smooth out any uneven areas but leave most of your existing base intact. Clean up any flakes of mascara and stale make-up residue under the eye by dipping the tip of a cotton bud in eye make-up remover and tracing it just beneath the lashes. Make sure the area is completely free of cleanser before applying any more make-up.

2 For a wonderful, luminous effect, dust the skin with a slightly iridescent powder. This will help light to bounce off tired skin, rejuvenating it at a stroke. And if you are changing into more revealing clothes, don't save it just for your face. Golden-toned powders also look great brushed lightly over the décolletage and collarbones.

3 Highlighting your bone structure will have a dramatic effect, so apply a stroke of shimmering, pearlized powder across your browbones and the tops of your cheekbones. Choose warm, creamy tones, which look more flattering on lacklustre skin than colder, silvery shades.

4 Dot a little gold or iridescent **pink powder** at the inner corner of the eye. This will have an instant **pick-me-up** effect without looking too heavy-handed.

5 Touch up any blemishes and dark shadows with concealer, but apply it with a brush so you **don't overdo it** or interfere with your existing make-up. And don't forget to **conceal any shadows** that have appeared at the very corners of your eyes by the bridge of the nose, a common occurrence at the end of **a long day.**

6 Mascara is a very obliging make-up tool, and **two coats** look better than one in the evening. You can apply a second coat over your existing **mascara,** provided you comb through the lashes **immediately** after applying it.

7 Pinky, coral-toned blushers bring a flush of **energy and vitality** to drained skin, which is always useful at the end of the day. For **evening**, try a slightly darker shade than you normally wear so that its effect is **visible** in evening light. Olive skins will benefit from a little **bronzing powder** dusted over the central panels of the cheeks.

8 Focus on either eyes or lips to **save time** and make your overall appearance look more refined. So go for **glamorous** deep red lips teamed with defined brows and **a hint of shine** on the browbone, or added definition around the eye. For a look that's **smoky and smouldering,** apply shadow all around the eye, as close to the base of the lashes as you can get it.

9 For **voluptuous** evening lips, try the old trick of using a **paler shade** at the centre of your mouth and a darker one towards the edge, but make sure you **blend them** well.

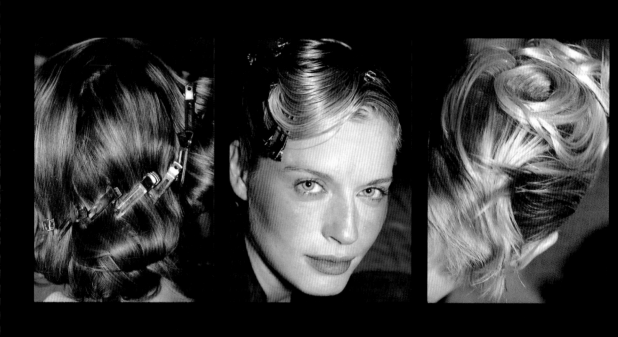

haircare

THE QUEST FOR

great HAIR

Our hair says more about us than any other feature. Its cut, colour and condition are all expressions of our personality and the image we choose to project and, while strong, shiny hair is one of the biggest confidence-boosters around, we all know that bad hair days – or cuts – can seriously dent our self-esteem.

Some psychologists believe that we attach labels to different hair colours, with blondes seen as passive, brunettes assertive, and redheads fiery and temperamental. But the truth is that everything about our hair makes a statement of some kind, whether it is long or short, natural or highly styled, soft or severe.

THE RIGHT CUT

The key to gorgeous hair is a good cut, and that means one that flatters the shape of your face and suits your hair type (for more information on both these aspects of haircare, turn to page 17). Take your lifestyle into account, too – some styles are much more time-consuming than others. And to maintain a great cut, remember the importance of regular trims. Not only will these make you look and feel good – a salon visit is a pampering experience, after all – they really are beneficial as they'll promote healthy hair and keep dry, broken ends in check.

If you are trying a new hairdresser, even one who has been recommended, ask for a consultation first. A good stylist will happily spend ten minutes or so talking to you before picking up the scissors, during which time you can get a feel for the salon and check out some of the finished cuts. Take pictures from magazines if you

Hair that's strong and healthy will really shine

are worried you won't be able to describe the look that you want, but be prepared for a realistic assessment of what will and won't work for your hair. It's far better to know in advance that a particular style won't suit you.

A trip to the salon should be a time for relaxation, but try to make the most of your hairdresser's expertise and ask questions while you are there. You can pick up drying and styling techniques that will work at home, as well as product recommendations. And if at any point you are unhappy with what you see, ask the stylist to stop and talk you through what he or she is doing. Equally, if you feel the slightest discomfort during a chemical treatment such as a perm or tint, get someone to check your hair straight away. Leaving the salon with a shorter cut than you expected is one thing; leaving with hair that has been damaged is quite another.

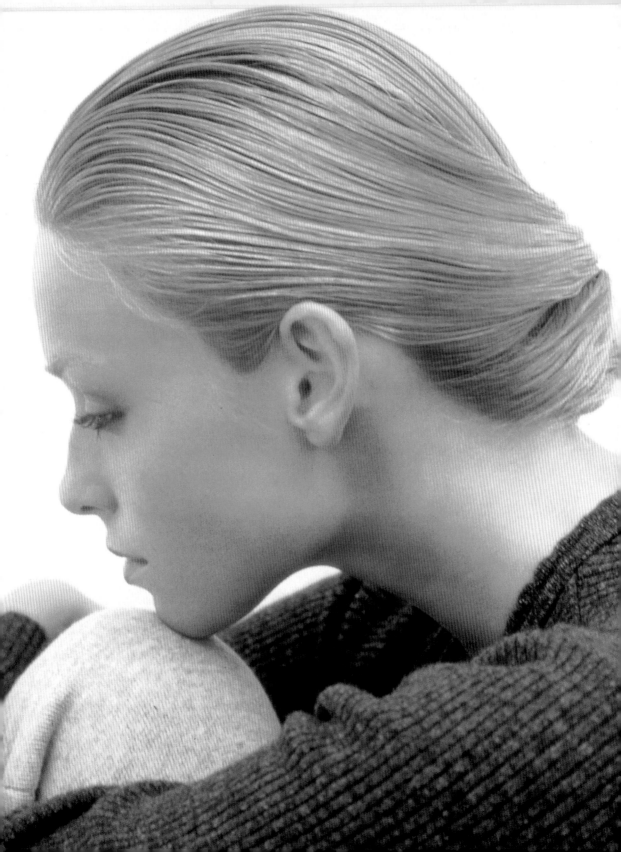

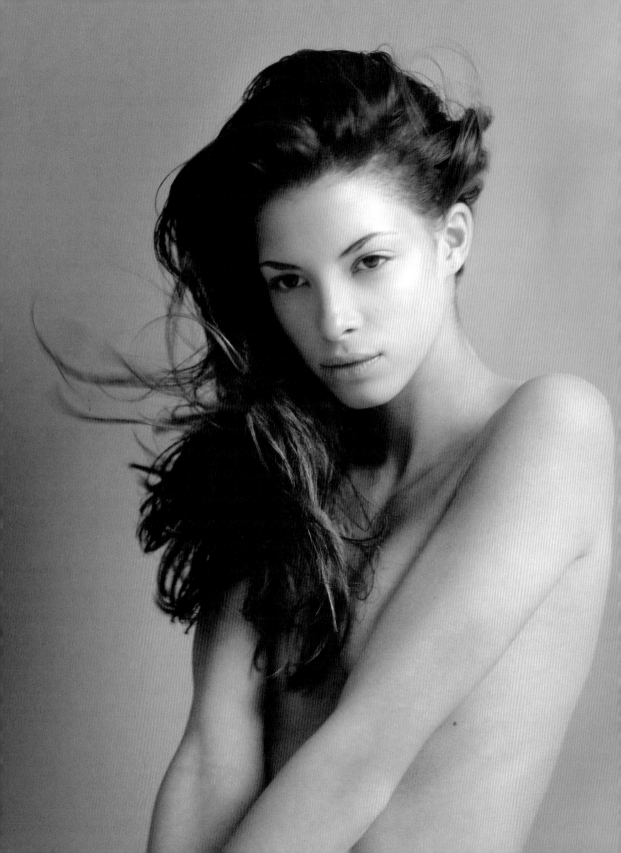

BACK TO BASICS – WHICH PRODUCTS DO YOU NEED?

We spend more money on haircare than we do on any other aspect of beauty, and the range of products available continues to grow. Shampoos, conditioners and therapeutic treatments have benefited hugely from recent scientific advances, and regular use of a few carefully chosen products will help keep your hair in optimum condition. But before you rush to the chemist or beauty counter, reconsider your hair type. A head of beautiful, healthy hair depends on the correct use of the right products over a sustained period of time, not a series of impulse buys.

Start with the basics. If you are using mismatched shampoos and conditioners, such as shampoo for oily hair and conditioner for normal, try to streamline your selection and take at least these two products from the same range and hair type. Choosing the right sort of conditioner is important, too. If you aren't sure which to go for, try combing your hair when you have just washed it. If it snags in the first few centimetres, the chances are that you need a heavyweight conditioner. If the comb makes it halfway through, you probably only need a detangler.

Be guided by your hair type. Hair that is chemically damaged, naturally dry or dehydrated by the sun will obviously need some extra help, but oily hair can also benefit from conditioner. If you find it makes your hair heavy or lank, try a lighter formula or just apply it to the ends.

Once you have the right products, make sure you get the most out of them. Many of us are guilty of overloading our hair with shampoo or conditioner, which makes it difficult to rinse. A blob the size of a 10p piece should be plenty and, if you really need more, it's better to repeat the process rather than slathering on too much in the first place.

Another common mistake is to forget that conditioners need time to work their magic. We may think we have left them on our hair for the required five minutes, but the truth is that we usually only give them about 45 seconds to impart their active ingredients, which isn't nearly long enough. And few of us spend enough time working them through the hair and over the scalp. When this is done by a professional, it feels like a head massage and this is what you should be aiming for at home. Even the best products can't work effectively if they don't come into contact with the hair itself.

Finally, the old trick of rinsing your hair under the cold tap after conditioning can really improve its appearance. Hair is made up of a central core or shaft which is encased in cuticles that overlap rather like tiles on a roof. While very hot water causes the cuticles to swell and stand away from the hair shaft, cold water makes them flatten against the central core, creating a smooth, shiny surface. Conditioners and other treatment products contribute to this process by filling tiny gaps between the cuticles and hair shaft that have been caused by rough handling, and by creating a light-reflective coating around the cuticles themselves.

REALIZE YOUR HAIR'S TRUE POTENTIAL

The technology that revolutionized skincare and make-up formulations has also transformed many haircare products. So instead of having to visit a salon for hair that's

The fragrance factor

Fragrance is a key factor when it comes to choosing hair products. Your hair is surprisingly effective at perfuming the air around you and, unless it's very short, will impart the scent of your shampoo and conditioner whenever you are on the move. Many delicious natural ingredients have been incorporated into haircare products. This is primarily for their therapeutic values – herbs such as rosemary and thyme add shine to dark hair, while coconut and orange oils have great moisturizing properties – but the fact that they smell lovely is an added bonus.

Alternatively, if your favourite fragrance is available in an alcohol-free formula (many now are), you can spray it lightly over your hair. It won't dry or damage it, but it will make you smell wonderful.

sleek, glossy and full of life, you can now achieve these looks at home.

Build volume Fine, flyaway hair is a problem for many women, so the very word volume is full of promise. But can it be delivered? Tongs and heated rollers used to be the only way to build air and height into a style, by creating body at the roots. And while those tricks still work, shampoos, conditioners and styling products have now been developed to inject volume into the hair itself.

Most of these work by depositing bulking ingredients, such as wheat proteins, under the cuticles, making the individual hairs look thicker. The effects of these products, which last from one wash to the next, are cumulative. So while a volumizing shampoo will make a difference, the combination of a volumizing shampoo, conditioner and styling spray will really transform your hair (turn to page 136 for a step-by-step guide to building volume into fine hair).

Mousses are another way of adding body, though they can be drying. For the best results, divide your hair into sections and apply the mousse close to the roots.

Add shine and hold The latest serums and clear, spritz-on polishing liquids will lock in moisture and add a lustrous sheen to dull hair, coating the strands with light-reflective, moisturizing ingredients as well as smoothing the cuticles to create an even finish. Gels, which are also effective holding agents, can be applied with your hands to wet hair and combed through. Use them sparingly but don't panic if you think you've overdone it. Simply rinse your comb and pass it through your hair again to remove the excess.

Waxes or pomades, which give a really slick look, can also be applied with your fingertips, but warm the product between your palms first so it's easy to spread through your hair. Wax is designed to give a textured look, separating individual strands of hair, so be sure to work it well into the ends (turn to page 138 to see how wax can be used to transform short hair).

Beware of heavy-handedness when using wax-based products – if you use too much, your hair will just look greasy. A very little goes a long way so start by dotting a tiny amount into your palms and see how you go. It's much easier to add more than it is to take away.

The importance of protection

- Most of us describe our hair as fine and fragile, yet we treat it as though it was the toughest, most resilient thing in the world. So handle it with care. Instead of dragging combs and brushes through it when it's wet, for example, pat it dry and then gently remove the tangles, working from the ends to the roots. Try to find a seamless comb – one that is moulded in one piece – so there are no jagged ridges to scrape the hair cuticles.
- Hairdryers and heated styling appliances are major culprits when it comes to damaging hair. If you feel your hair really needs a heated blast, leave it to dry naturally for a while if you can, and give it a final burst with the dryer. The moment when heat actively helps hold a style comes at the end of the drying process, so this should be all you need.
- Be careful with tongs and crimpers. If yours are covered with little black spots, you've probably singed your hair and damaged the cuticles, so apply one of the latest protective styling products, such as a conditioning serum.
- Don't forget that hair, like skin, can be damaged by the sun. Protect it in summer, whatever its type, with hair oils and spritzes that screen out the harmful UV rays.

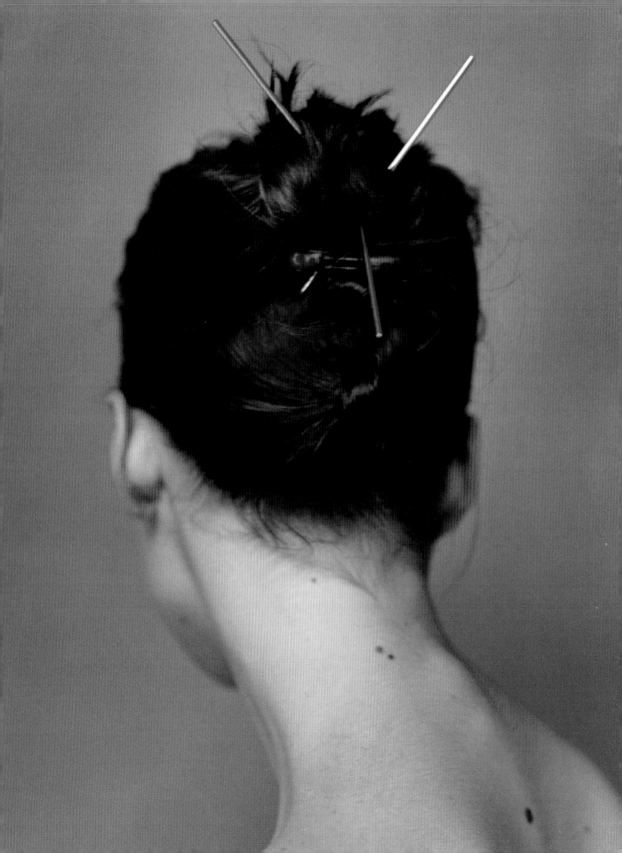

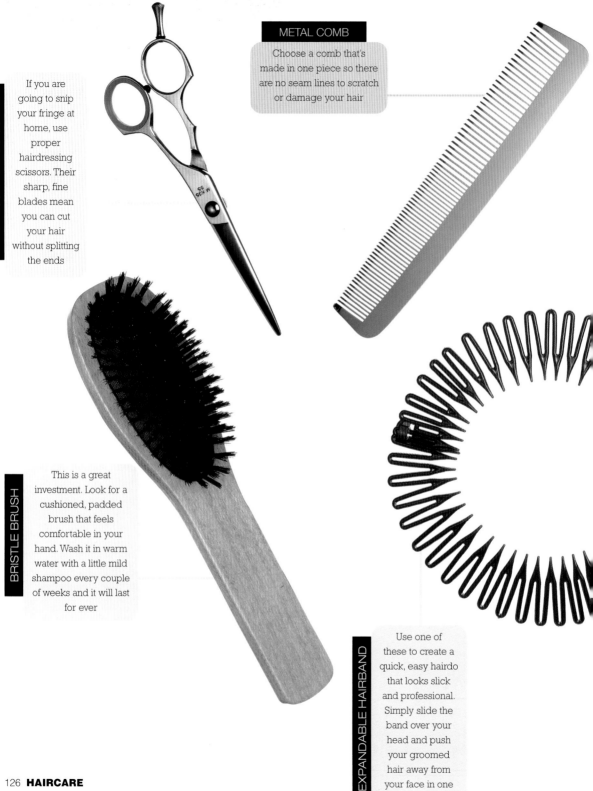

Choose a comb that's made in one piece so there are no seam lines to scratch or damage your hair

PROFESSIONAL SCISSORS

If you are going to snip your fringe at home, use proper hairdressing scissors. Their sharp, fine blades mean you can cut your hair without splitting the ends

BRISTLE BRUSH

This is a great investment. Look for a cushioned, padded brush that feels comfortable in your hand. Wash it in warm water with a little mild shampoo every couple of weeks and it will last for ever

EXPANDABLE HAIRBAND

Use one of these to create a quick, easy hairdo that looks slick and professional. Simply slide the band over your head and push your groomed hair away from your face in one smooth movement

know-how

Much of the damage we inflict on our hair is caused by rough handling and poorly designed tools. A basic kit of inexpensive, hair-friendly essentials should solve these problems

ELASTIC BANDS

These snag-free elastic bands are flatter than most, so they won't cut into your hair. If you can't get hold of them, make your own with lengths of haberdashers' elastic

SILVER CLIPS

Snap-shut clips like these will secure your hair more effectively than hairgrips, making it easier to dry in sections or to keep off your face when applying make-up

HOOK-END ELASTICS

Tugging a ponytail through a circular band can pull your hair and mess up your bunch, but these elastics will hook into your hair and can then be wound around to hold it securely

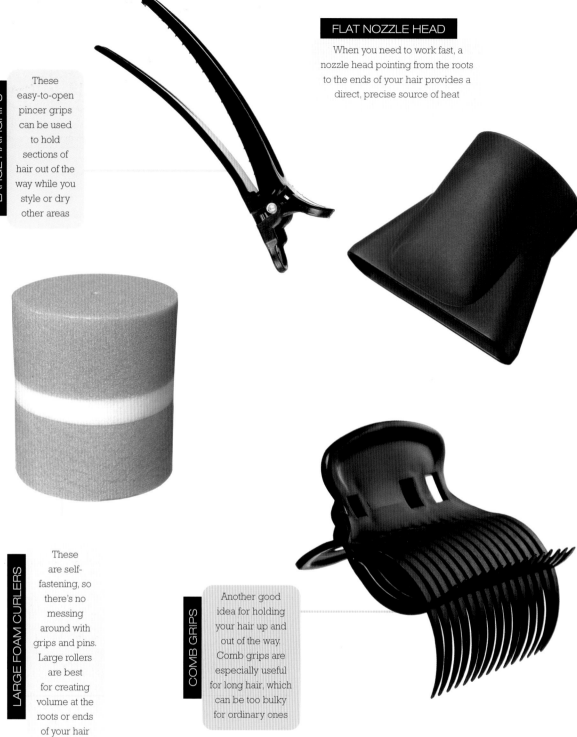

These easy-to-open pincer grips can be used to hold sections of hair out of the way while you style or dry other areas

FLAT NOZZLE HEAD

When you need to work fast, a nozzle head pointing from the roots to the ends of your hair provides a direct, precise source of heat

These are self-fastening, so there's no messing around with grips and pins. Large rollers are best for creating volume at the roots or ends of your hair

Another good idea for holding your hair up and out of the way. Comb grips are especially useful for long hair, which can be too bulky for ordinary ones

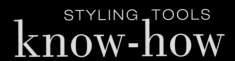

STYLING TOOLS
know-how

One of the keys to successful styling is using the right appliance for the look you hope to achieve. Brushes, nozzles, clips and combs can all make a difference to the finished result

BARREL BRUSH

This is an extremely useful styling tool, which enables you to grip and pull your hair straight as you blow-dry it

DIFFUSER HEAD

These deliver gentle heat, which gives you more time to style your hair. The prongs can also be used to fluff and lift the hair

STRAIGHTENING IRONS

These are great for a super-sleek evening look. They can even benefit straight hair by flattening split ends and new hairs, and straightening crinkly ones. Solid irons will also transform curly hair

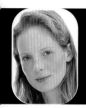

DRY, FRIZZY
HAIR

see page 21

Hair like Arabella's may seem hard to handle but with the right products and techniques, it really is possible to **transform dry frizz** into smooth, shiny hair. **Regular trims** should be a priority to avoid split ends and keep your hair in good condition, and it's also important to choose products with **UV filters** to protect it from the drying effects of the sun.

Resist the temptation to towel-dry hair after washing as this will disturb its surface cuticles, making it feel coarse and even drier. Instead, **pat it dry** with a towel. And never yank a comb through wet hair – it will make it stretch and then crinkle. For a really **rich, moisturizing** treatment, slick some olive oil on to towel-patted hair, wrap in a towel and leave for about 45 minutes. Remove with a light shampoo for **shiny, highly conditioned locks.** For evenings, try smoothing your hair with straightening irons to tame frizzy, broken ends, but apply a heat-protective serum first.

avoid

volumizing shampoos and conditioners

alcohol-based sprays and mousses, which can be drying

look for

sculpting gels and serums

fabric-covered elastic bands, which won't damage hair

alcohol-free styling products

CUTS THAT WORK

One-length cuts emphasize the problems of dry hair, especially if it's long. Gentle layers, on the other hand, will create a softer silhouette and minimize dryness at the ends. They will also help the hair to form curls rather than frizz.

COLOURS TO TRY

Vegetable dyes and natural plant-based colours are ideal for drier hair types as they deliver high shine and colour with none of the chemical stress of peroxide- or ammonia-based dyes.

STYLING TIPS

Take advantage of the frizz-taming products now available. Leave-in serums can be spread through your hair to create a smooth surface, but use them sparingly. On really bad frizz days, use a little wet-look gel or pomade to smooth the hair into a side-parted crop, a sleek bob that tucks behind your ears or a French pleat.

TIP Use conditioning serums only where you need them to avoid oily roots. Work them through the ends of your hair first, and finish by smoothing them over the surface

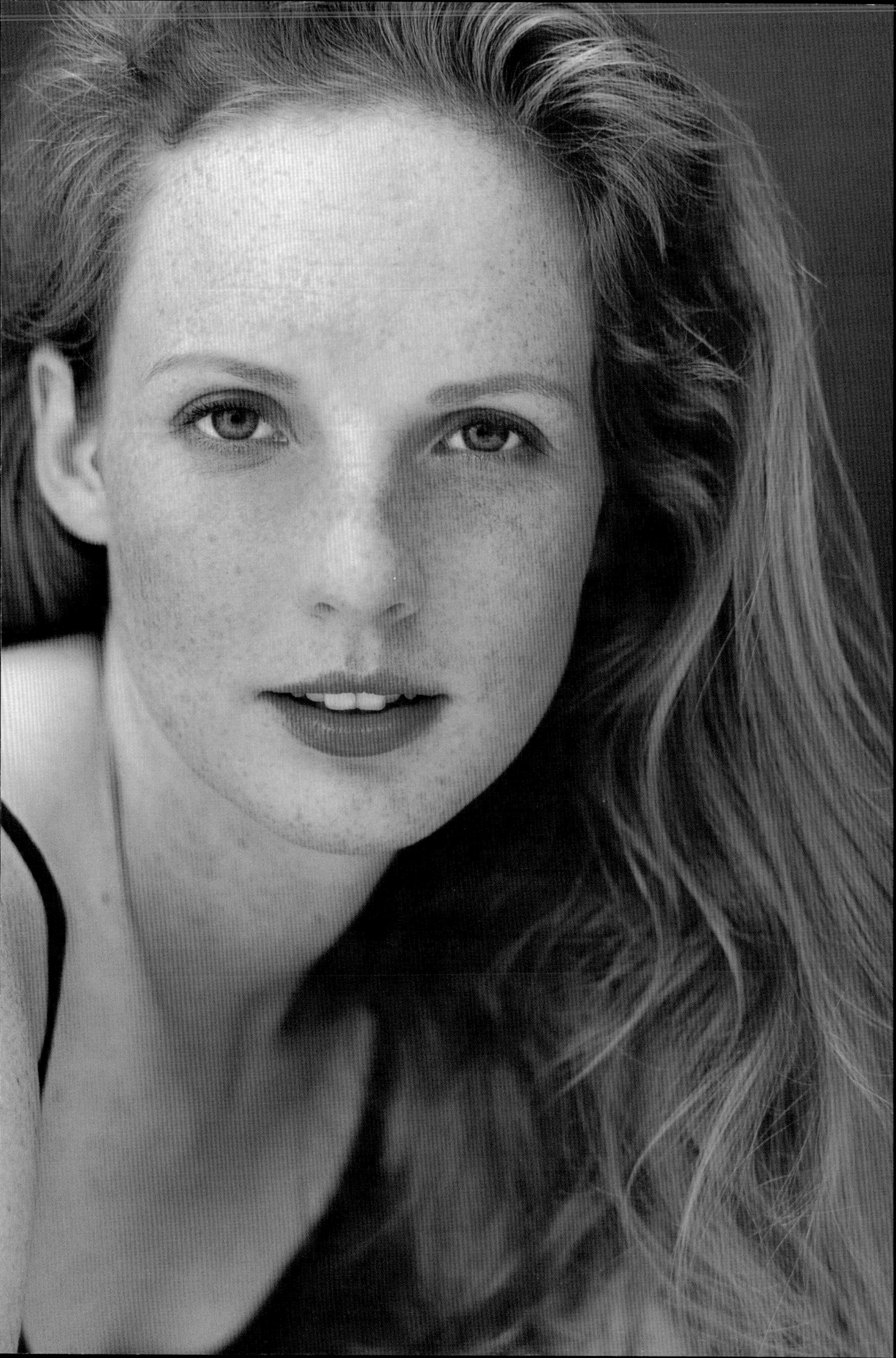

real hair

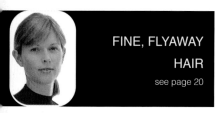

FINE, FLYAWAY
HAIR
see page 20

Fine hair like Jo's is almost always very straight and, although this can cause problems, it is usually easy to keep in good condition. So once you have added body and got your flyaway locks under control, you should have a super-sleek head of hair. Length is an obstacle for fine hair. It simply doesn't have the weight to break over the shoulders and will tend to sit there a little forlornly, so stick to shoulder-length styles. Graduated, layered cuts, described below, not only look great but can also be used to help lift the hair at the roots, where it can look rather flat.

Frequent washing can be self-defeating for fine hair as it tends to be more flyaway than ever when it's freshly washed. If you leave it for a day or two, however, it looks and feels more bulky. Volumizing mousses will create the 'root lift' associated with thicker hair if they are applied to this area only, while the hairdressers' trick of drying the hair upside down can also help.

avoid

heavy conditioners – they'll make
your hair even more limp
nylon brushes and combs, which can
exacerbate any static problems

look for

anti-static conditioners, which give extra hold

volumizing shampoos and mousses, to add body

glaze liquids, which give hair a glassy sheen

CUTS THAT WORK

Cuts that build graduated layers into the hair will make it seem thicker. Wedge shapes and blunt bobs also work well, giving swing and movement to fine hair. Avoid choppy, textured cuts as your hair won't hold them well. Instead, go for styles that will emphasize sleekness and shine while adding volume.

COLOURS TO TRY

Colour can be used to great effect on fine hair. Lowlights and highlights will add depth, giving the illusion of extra body and volume, while solid colour rinses enhance fine, straight hair by emphasizing its shine.

STYLING TIPS

When you apply mousse to add volume, separate your hair into sections to make sure you get the product close to the roots. Use a diffuser head on your hairdryer and push its small prongs into the hair to intensify the body-building process.

TIP Apply hairspray by spraying it on to your hairbrush and then brushing your hair. This will ensure a light, even distribution and a natural-looking finish

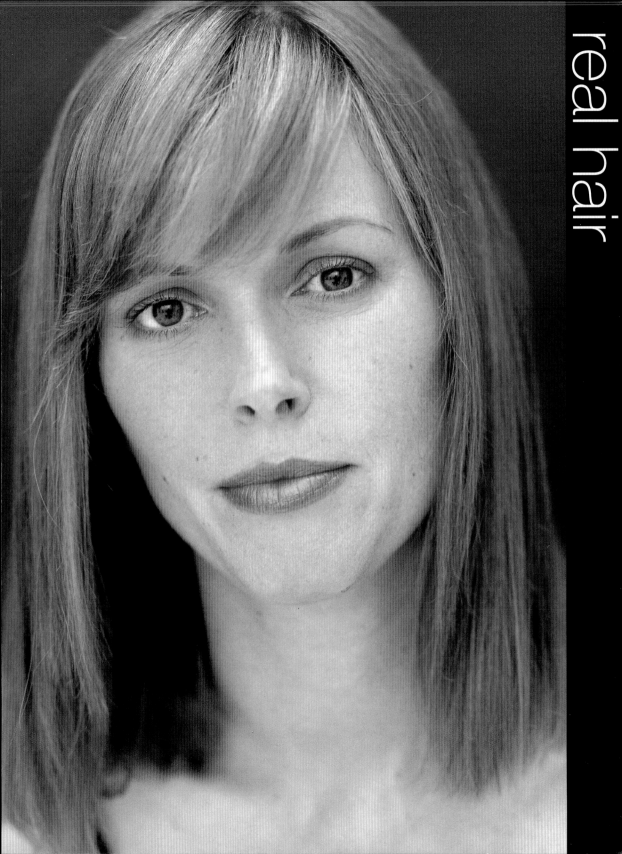

real hair

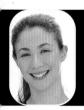

OILY, LANK
HAIR

see page 21

Oily hair like Susanna's is an inherited problem and, like oily skin, it's highly influenced by **hormonal activity** in the body. Harsh products that **strip out** the hair's natural oils definitely aren't the answer – they'll simply encourage the scalp's oil-producing glands to compensate by **going into overdrive**. Anti-dandruff shampoos can be aggressive, too, so if you suffer from dandruff, try massaging a couple of drops of tea tree oil into your scalp instead.

Oily hair shouldn't be washed in very hot water as this will trigger yet more oil production. Use **lukewarm water** and, if you can face it, blast your hair with cold water after your final rinse. Many conditioners are **too rich** for oily hair but if yours really needs one, choose a lightweight formula and apply it to the ends only. Go easy with heated appliances, too. Overbrushing and playing with your hair will encourage oil production, so try to **leave it alone** – tie it back during the day if you can't help touching it.

avoid

stress – it can trigger oil production

creamy conditioners

overworking your hair, which

stimulates oil production

look for

mild, frequent-use shampoos

lightweight spray-in conditioners, to detangle

styling mousses, to build volume

CUTS THAT WORK

Excess oil can leave your hair lank and lifeless, and one-length cuts can make things worse. Try chunky layers, which will add body and movement. Layers have an added bonus for oily hair – they lift the strands themselves away from the roots, allowing air to circulate and preventing oil from travelling down the hair shaft.

COLOURS TO TRY

Lowlights and highlights are a good idea if you have lank, greasy hair. Their slight bleaching action will make your hair a little drier, and they'll also break up the mono-tone shades that seem to make oily roots particularly obvious.

STYLING TIPS

Finger-drying the roots of your hair will avoid overheating the oily area, as well as creating lift and volume. Remember to keep your styling tools, brushes and combs scrupulously clean by washing them once a week in lukewarm water and with a little mild shampoo.

TIP To prevent heat-damage, apply a little leave-in conditioner to the ends of your hair before styling. This will protect and nourish the ends without exacerbating oily roots

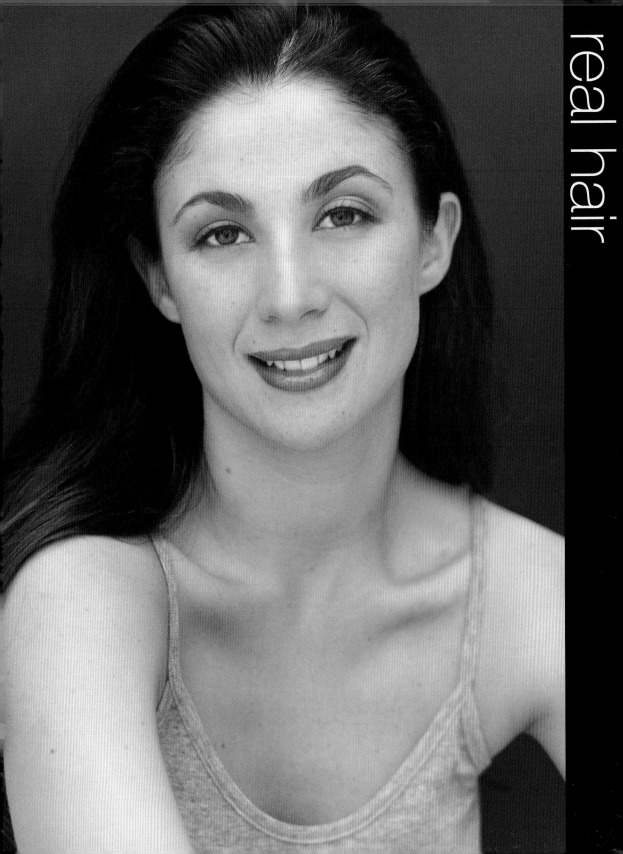

real hair

HOW TO
blow-dry
your hair

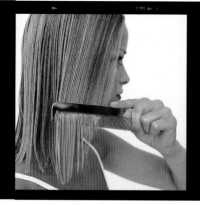

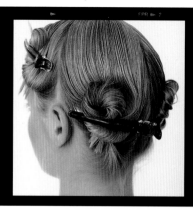

Recreate the sleek finish of
professionally blow-dried
hair with these simple steps

1 Shampoo and condition your
hair, then towel-dry. Using a
fine-toothed comb, remove all knots
and tangles. Apply any heat-protective
styling products at this point.

2 Divide your hair into three or four
sections. This may take a few
minutes but it does mean you can
concentrate on one area at a time
rather than trying to cope with your
whole head of hair at once, which can
be difficult to manage. Clip unwanted
sections out of the way.

HOW TO
add volume to
fine hair

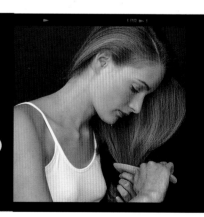

Even fine, lank hair can be given
body and bounce with the
right products and techniques

1 Wash your hair with a
volumizing shampoo and
conditioner, then towel-dry. Lightly
apply a volumizing styling spray or
gel, then divide your hair into rough
sections. Always check that any
products you apply are suitable for
use with heated appliances.

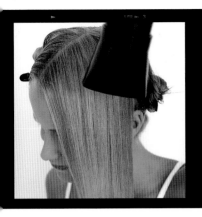
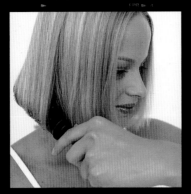

3 Use a flat nozzle on the end of your hairdryer to direct heat exactly where you want it. Next, take a roller brush. Brush one section of hair from the roots to the tips, then roll your hair around the brush and, with your dryer in the other hand, gently pull it taut. This action gives professionally blow-dried hair its lovely swing.

4 Work around your whole head, rolling the sections of hair over the brush and holding it taut under the dryer. Finish by turning your head upside down and giving the roots a quick blast of warm air. Then simply brush through for ultra-sleek locks.

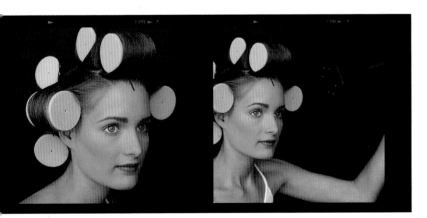

2 Take a set of large foam rollers. Wind one hair section around one of the rollers. Next, curl the ends of your hair over, then under, the roller before rolling up – you should finish with the top part of the hair section over the roller. Repeat with the remaining sections of hair.

3 Dry your hair slowly using a diffuser, which will ensure a steady flow of warm air. When your hair is dry, unwind the rollers. Turn your head upside down, spritz your hair lightly with styling spray, then gently brush it through, holding the ends as you brush them.

HOW TO
create a
French pleat

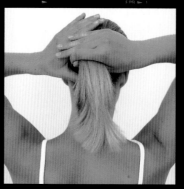

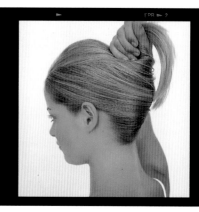

The classic chignon, which always looks chic and elegant, is quick and easy to achieve

1 This look works well on long or mid-length hair. Start by brushing your hair, then hold it as if in a bunch at the back of your head, at about the height of your orbital bone (the bumpy bit that sticks out).

2 Grasp the hair close to your head and slowly slide your hands down to the ends, gently twisting it as you go. As you reach the ends, turn the twist of hair into your head, bringing the ends up towards your crown.

HOW TO
transform a
textured crop

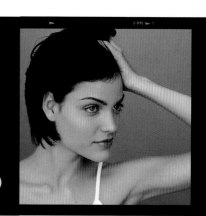

A gamine crop can be dressed up for evenings with a slick of pomade and a sparkly hairgrip

1 Take a tiny blob of pomade or polishing product and warm it between the palms of your hands. Choose a pomade with a little sparkle if you want to look really dramatic. Work the product through your hair, from the roots to the tips.

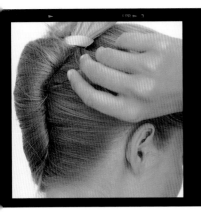

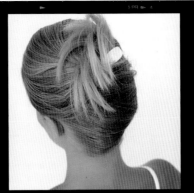

3 Secure the top of the twisted hair to the crown area with a decorative clip. Then pin the twist on the folded-over side to the back of your head with hairgrips.

4 Finally, spray your fingers with a little hairspray and use them to smooth the sides of your hair. Once you have tamed any wisps with spray, flatten or tuck them into the French pleat itself.

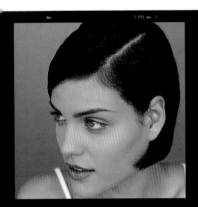

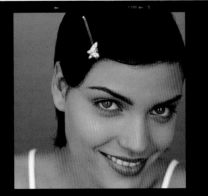

2 Next, take a fine-toothed comb and part your hair about three-quarters of the way across your forehead. Smooth the hair on either side of the parting with a comb and the palm of your hand.

3 Finish, if you like, by adding a hair accessory to the wider front section. A diamanté or tortoiseshell clip in your fringe will create a very gamine look.

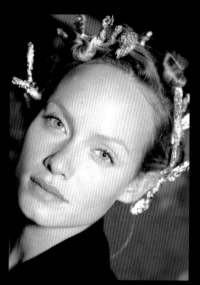
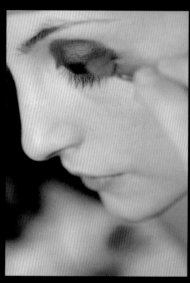
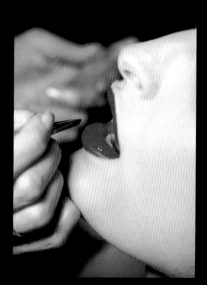

beauty
solutions

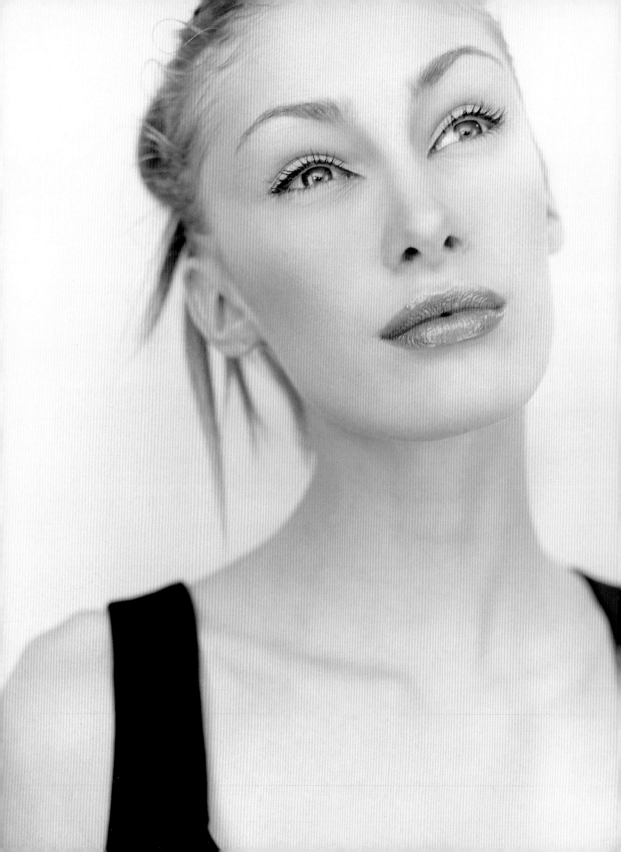

shop
TALK

Beauty shopping can be a daunting experience. Quite simply, there is so much choice that it's not surprising we sometimes make mistakes. Even the experts buy the wrong things from time to time.

Of the make-up personalities described in this book, hoarders are the most likely to make impulse buys, which is why they often end up with drawers full of barely used lipsticks and eyeshadows at home. Beauty eclectics are also prone to making unwise purchases – they find it hard to put together a coherent make-up collection as so many things appeal to them. If this applies to you, next time you go shopping for a practical, matt foundation, try to ignore the pearly iridescent ones, however eyecatching they may be.

The other beauty personalities are better able to cope with the dazzling array of goodies on show at the beauty counters. The minimalist knows exactly what she wants and prides herself on her pared-down make-up kit, while the woman who lives in the past only ventures out to replace her tried-and-tested favourites.

For most of us, though, the problem is the bewildering array of products available. And it's worth remembering that although counter assistants are there to help and advise you, they are also there to sell their products, as many as they can. This can make it difficult to escape with only one item. Unexpected special offers are an added temptation, but the shrewd shopper only succumbs to these when they include products she really needs. So unless this is the case, steer clear of promotions and stick to your original shopping list. Trial sizes and samples are a far better way of experimenting with new things, especially as they are often free.

A FRESH APPROACH

If you are feeling brave and don't mind having your face made up in the middle of a department store, why not try a makeover? This is a great way to have your make-up applied by someone with professional skills and a totally fresh eye, free of charge. It also means you can try colours and textures you may never have considered, without having to buy a thing.

The down side is that you may feel obliged to make a hefty purchase at the end of the session. Don't be. Before you sit down, promise yourself that you won't buy anything straight away. Instead, get the assistant to record all the colours and products she has used – most companies have illustrated faces to show what went where that you can take away with you. This means you can reassess the colours in daylight, see how the products last and find out what your friends think of them.

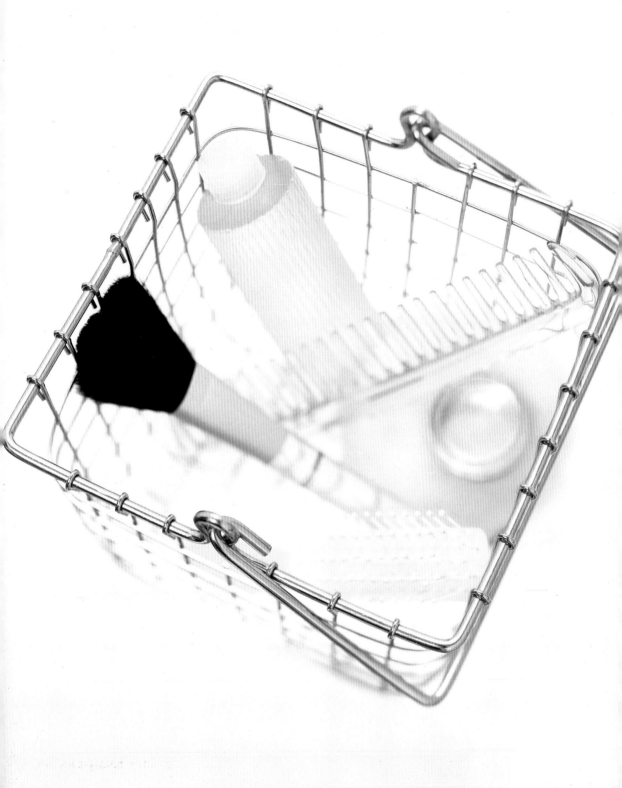

BEAUTY ON THE SHELF

Shopping at stand-alone counters is an ideal way to try new things. Confident shoppers will feel free to try the colours on display without the watchful eye of the counter assistant, while beauty novices are more likely to experiment if they can do so without having to ask for help. Remember, however, that these aren't the best places to buy foundation. Many beauty houses will let you fill a sample pot with enough foundation for several days if you talk to the sales staff, so make the most of this opportunity and treat yourself to a proper home trial before your next purchase.

Before you buy any skincare products, make sure you have a basic understanding of your own skin. Even if you aren't exactly sure of your skin type, you know much more about it than anyone else and the important thing is that you communicate its characteristics accurately. Everyone's skin is different – yours may be essentially oily but dry on the surface; normally clear but prone to unexpected breakouts; usually well-behaved but showing signs of becoming sensitive, so take all these things into account. Refer to the sections in this book on skin analysis (page 15) and care (page 24) for more guidance.

Less is usually more with skincare, so don't go mad and buy every product in a range. Start with one or two and see how your skin gets on with them. And stick to the smaller sizes to begin with – you can always trade up to the larger ones later. Lastly, remember that any new regime should be given a reasonable trial period. Give new products a good month, provided they don't trigger a negative reaction, before you assess their strengths and weaknesses.

Testing make-up colours

- Keep a clean sheet of paper in your bag for testing new lip colours, especially if you are buying one to go with a particular outfit. Swatches of eyeshadow can be made in the same way, giving you the chance to check the colours in daylight, away from the pressure of the beauty counters.
- The coverage of a foundation can often be judged by its pouring consistency, so tip tester bottles gently to see how the liquid flows. Thinner, faster-flowing products tend to produce lighter, less intense coverage.
- Remember that the best way to judge a foundation is to try it on your face. That's where the colour is actually going to be worn, after all. If you are already wearing foundation, the best alternatives are your neck or your inner arm. Hands tend to be a little darker in tone than faces, so using these as a guide is sure to lead to a mismatch.
- Artificial light is the biggest problem in any shop. In fact, it makes it almost impossible to assess the true colour of a foundation, which means finding the right match for your skin is equally difficult. In most department stores, however, the cosmetic areas are on the ground floor near the doors, so the best thing to do is to apply a little foundation and go outside to check the colour in daylight.
- Most companies now offer small pots of nail polish, which are great for the season's hot, new colours. The bigger pots are better for classic neutral shades, which may be less dramatic but are more subtle and versatile – this is what makes them such a valuable part of your year-round make-up kit.

BEAUTY
problem
SOLVING

I suffer from really puffy eyes. Is there a quick fix for this?

Ridding yourself of puffy eyes at the last minute isn't something you should do every day but, in a real emergency, try chilling two teaspoons in the fridge. Then hold them, hollow sides down, over your closed eyes for a few seconds. If you have a little more time, steep two camomile teabags in boiled water, leave them to cool and then place them over your eyes for a few minutes.

I have noticed red patches developing on my cheeks. They are also a little bumpy. What could they be caused by?

This sounds like acne rosacea, a form of acne that is more common among women than men as their skin is finer and more delicate. As with all forms of acne, you should consult your GP as soon as possible. He or she will be able to prescribe mild antibiotics that should prevent the condition from getting worse. Stronger antibiotics, now widely available for more severe forms of acne, are extremely successful if they are taken soon enough.

Is there a simple way to work out whether I have warm or cool skin tones?

Hold a good-sized piece of silver paper or fabric up to your face, then do the same with a gold piece. Warm skin tones will sit best with the gold paper while cool ones will be flattered by the silver. It's worth establishing which of these two descriptions applies to your skin as it will help you choose the right make-up colours. Red/orange-based shades work well with warm skin tones; cooler ones look best with red/blue-based shades.

I have recently developed sensitive, itchy skin. Why is this?

If your skin has only recently shown signs of irritation, and you haven't changed your skincare routine, check out your perfume. It could be that this is causing an allergic reaction, making your skin itchy and sensitive. Food allergies, central heating and air conditioning are also potential skin irritants so, if possible, try a process of elimination to identify the source of your problems.

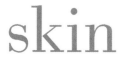

skin

features

How can I tell if my make-up gives equal emphasis to my features?

Try to stand back and take a good look at yourself. For the sake of accuracy, we tend to apply make-up right up close to a mirror, but this makes it difficult to get an overall view. Assessing yourself from a distance will help you to see if you are drawing too much attention certain features at the expense of others.

I have a small mouth. How can I use make-up techniques to make it look bigger?

Rather than overemphasizing your lips with liner to create a fuller-looking pout, try Marilyn Monroe's trick of wearing graduated shades of the same colour. She reputedly wore five shades of red, but two shades of lip colour will do fine. Apply the darker colour at the outer edge, as far into the lip line as you can without it looking unnatural. Then apply the paler shade in the centre of your lips. Finally, dab a little gloss right in the centre. This will give the impression of plumping up the lips, but with no heavy lines.

I have a very poorly defined chin and jawline. Is there anything I can do about it?

There are plenty of things you can do about this problem. Having your hair cut in a jaw-length bob that falls forward will help create definition and shadow in this area, as well as providing a line between the face and neck. You can draw attention to your mouth by using bold lip colours or, if you really don't want to emphasize this area, go for smouldering eye make-up and make your eyes the focus of your face.

There are a few make-up techniques that you can try but keep them for evening use, and only then if you are very careful. Dab a little dusty-rose blusher under your chin and work in a V-shape from this central point out to the sides. Blend with a little transparent powder if the effect looks too strong. Sweep a little highlighter in an upside-down crescent over the centre of your chin. This works because pale shades bring things forward while darker shades make them appear to recede.

Are there any make-up tricks I can try to change the shape of my nose?

Sculpting your nose with shadows to make it seem slimmer is fine for models and actresses, but not such a good idea for everyday use. It can emphasize any grey shadows in the area and make the lighter central panel or bridge of the nose look broader. One trick that is worth a try is a light flick of beige/rose blush under the very tip, which will appear to shorten a very long nose.

My eyes really slope down at the edges, which means I always look tired. Is there anything I can do to rectify this?

With the right make-up techniques, you can 'lift' your eyes convincingly, so don't even think about surgery. Flicking your eyeliner up slightly at the outer corners of your eyes creates a strong lifting effect, while curling just your outer lashes before applying mascara to the whole lot is another effective trick. Finally, when you pluck your eyebrows, take slightly more hairs from beneath the outer edges than the inner ones. This will also give the impression of lifting your eyes.

How can I grow my fringe out without looking absolutely awful in the meantime?

Growing out a fringe can be an extremely painful process. Try layering the fringe and add a few more layers to the sides of your hair to blend it in. Alternatively, slick it back with a little gel and hold it away from your face with a skinny, modern headband.

One side of my hair rolls under as it should, but the other always kinks outwards. What can I do?

It sounds strange but the best way to deal with this problem is to use a roller brush and dry the hair outwards at the ends while it is still fairly damp. Then reverse the brush and pull the hair back under as it goes from damp to dry. This will reinforce the curl and help counter the hair's natural desire to kink outwards. If you don't want to blow-dry your hair, try using a few soft, foam curlers on the problem side while you sleep.

Styling products always seem to make my hair heavy. Am I using them incorrectly?

You are probably applying them unevenly and too liberally. If you are using gel or serum, start with a blob the size of a 10p piece. You can use a little more mousse, but dot small quantities throughout your hair instead of one large amount. Always squeeze styling products into your palms first, then smooth them between your hands before actually taking them through your hair.

I'm bored with my hair. What can I do?

Getting bored with your hair suggests that it's time for a change of salon. It's easy to get stuck in a rut and keep the same style, but a fresh approach can mean a completely new look for you and your hair.

Colour is another option. With more semi-permanent shades and techniques around, colour doesn't necessarily lead to a huge commitment, and it can transform your hair. Don't forget that a change of hair colour may also mean a change of make-up, so be prepared for a total overhaul.

Somebody suggested talcum powder as a remedy for greasy hair. Is this a good idea?

The old trick of shaking a little talcum powder into greasy hair to disguise excess oil is only ever advisable if you have naturally blonde or dark blonde hair. Brunettes should steer clear of talc as it gives the hair a greyish look. A better idea is to smooth your hair into a ponytail or slick style that won't emphasize the grease.

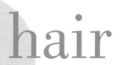

hair

make-up

Can I alter my lip colour without removing it?

If your lipstick suddenly strikes you as too loud but you don't have another shade to hand, try dotting a tiny amount of concealer over your lips, then press them together to mix the colours. This softens the colour quickly and effectively.

How do I get glossy lipstick to stay on?

For a long-lasting, glossy effect, try using lip pencil and clear gloss as an alternative to high-shine lipstick. Fill the entire lip area with lip pencil and apply the gloss over the top. This will help it stick to your lips.

If I make a mistake with my base, concealer or eye make-up, should I start again or can I tone down the errors?

It's not always necessary to start from scratch if you make a mistake. If you've overdone the concealer, simply dampen your fingers or a cotton bud with either water or saliva and use to wipe the surface gently. You can do the same for foundation, but use a damp sponge instead of a cotton bud. Water will remove some but not all of the make-up, unlike an oil-based cleanser. Use the same technique to tone down harshly applied eyeliner. And to correct heavy-handed eyeshadow application, use a clean, dry cotton-wool pad or a fluffy powder paddle brush (which has a downy surface rather than bristles) to dust the surface gently and lift away excess colour.

I always mess up my make-up when I apply mascara. How can I avoid this?

To avoid smudging mascara on your skin as you brush it on your lower lashes, place a mirror flat on a table top and look down into it as you apply the mascara. This increases the space between your lashes and your skin and, at the same time, allows you to work the mascara brush more freely.

My lipstick always bleeds into the fine lines around my mouth. Can I stop this?

A light layer of lip salve applied around your mouth, but not on your lips, is an effective way of preventing lipstick from feathering. The waxy oils in the salve will seal the area around the lips, creating a barrier and stopping the colour seeping over the edge.

My eyeliner line is always wonky. What can I do to create a more even finish?

For an even and well-defined line, pull the skin at the very edges of the eye gently outwards to make the lid itself as smooth as possible. Then work from the outside in rather than from the inner corner out. This will help you to create a smooth, fine, flowing line.

MAKE-UP IN
minutes

Modern lives rarely allow for time-consuming hair and make-up routines, but there's no need to spend hours in front of a mirror. With the right kit and a few professional hints, you can look sleek and groomed in a matter of minutes.

ten-minute make-up

Face Take a little time to apply and blend your concealer thoroughly, but instead of meticulously applying foundation, sweep translucent powder over your entire face to keep shine at bay.

Eyes A basic taupe eyeshadow is essential. Use it to cover the upper eyelid, concentrating the colour in the eye crease. Alternatively, use a muted eyeliner pencil – preferably grey or mid-brown – to draw around the eye, both above and below. Blend the edges gently with your fingertip, then finish with a single coat of mascara. If you have time, use an eyelash curler – a firm squeeze lasting just a couple of seconds will make a difference.

Lips Apply a coat of lip balm, then fill in the whole area with a lip pencil. This means you don't have to mess around with brushes and a multitude of different products, but leaves beautifully defined lips.

five-minute make-up

Face It may sound like an impossibly short time, but you can achieve plenty in five minutes. First, moisturize your skin, then take time to apply concealer. If you do this carefully, your face will look made-up even before any colour is applied. Face a good source of light, such as a window, so you don't have to waste time rechecking what you've already done.

Lips and brows Dark lip colours take too long to apply, so slick some clear or lightly coloured gloss across your lips. Then dab an eyebrow brush in a little of the same gloss and brush it through each eyebrow – brows are one of the keys to a well-groomed look.

Eyelashes Slick a coat of mascara over your lashes and comb through.

Cheeks and eyes Your moisturizer will now be absorbed, so apply your blusher. Sweep your brush in the blusher and, using rounded strokes, apply it over the apples of your cheeks. Then dust the same brush lightly over your eyelids and browbones. This will ensure your make-up looks complete.

one-minute make-up

All-in-one face Even one minute is time enough to treat your face to an injection of colour if you have the right tools. Chunky make-up sticks are great for lips, cheeks and eyes, and a muted rosy shade will be the most versatile. First, draw a line close to your eyelashes and blend it upwards with your fingertips. Dot a little on your cheeks and blend with your fingers. Finally, line your lips and fill with colour – this will take just a few seconds.

Quick kit: day

Lip Gloss Lightly coloured or clear.
Taupe eyeshadow A vital mid-tone.
Rose-coloured blush Good for virtually all skin tones and situations.
Chunky all-in-one make-up pencil A wise investment, and one that's easily transportable.

Quick kit: evening

Shimmering bronzing powder An essential staple that's quick and easy to use. Swept over your cheekbones, temples, shoulders and décolletage, this brings the skin to life in evening light.
Lip shines More pearlized than glossy, these can be dabbed on quickly using fingertips and still look fantastic.
Volumizing or iridescent mascara The one make-up element needed to dramatize eyes, mascara only takes seconds to apply.

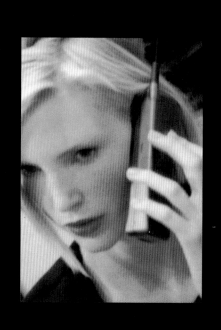

directory

Mail-order services

The following companies will send beauty products by post. Contact the numbers given for catalogues and delivery details.

Applewoods Retail Limited

Freepost 40 LON8989

London W1E 7BX

tel 0800-252322

fax 020-7487 2519

Traditional toiletries, soaps and bath oils.

L'Artisan Parfumeur

17 Cale Street

London SW3 3QR

tel 020-7352 4196

fax 020-7610 5317

http://www.mkn.co.uk/help/perfume/info

Fragrance specialists who also offer vouchers and a gift-wrapping service. Samples available.

Aveda

Avd Cosmetics

7 Munton Road

London SE17 1PR

tel 020-7410 1668

Great range of organically made cosmetics, skin- and haircare products.

Avon Cosmetics

3 Earlstress Road

Corby

Northamptonshire NN17 4AZ

tel 0845-605400

fax 01536-402493

http://www.uk.avon.com

A classic collection of innovative, affordable products, many containing the latest hi-tech ingredients.

Beauty Quest

Vestry Road

Sevenoaks

Kent TN14 5XA

tel 0541-505000

fax 01732-453166

Professional ranges devised by top make-up artists and hairdressers, plus well-known names including Aveda and Face Stockholm, and a selection of hair and beauty accessories.

Beauty World Direct

43 Market Place House

Market Place

Henley-on-Thames

Oxfordshire RG9 2AA

tel 0845-6000039

fax 01628-781301

Globally sourced beauty tools, including designer hair brushes from Paris, professional nailcare kit and American teeth-whitening systems.

Benefit

Benefit Counter

Selfridges

400 Oxford Street

London W1A 1AB

tel 020-7629 1234

Skincare and cosmetic products from San Francisco.

Charles H. Fox

22 Tavistock Street

London WC2E 7PY

tel 020-7240 3111

Suppliers to the film, TV and theatre worlds, but make-up and tools are also available to the general public.

Le Club des Créateurs de Beauté

Freepost LS5952

Parliament House

Parliament Terrace

Harrogate

North Yorkshire HG1 5BR

tel 0800-111315 (catalogues);

0990-902090 (order line)

fax 0990-903090

http://www.createurs-debeaute.com

French company that offers cosmetics by Agnès b, skincare by Professor Jean Cotte and Michel Klein perfumes.

Cosmetics à la Carte

102 Avro House

Havelock Terrace

London SW8 4AS

tel/fax 020-7622 2318

http://www.a-la-carte.co.uk

Cosmetic specialists offering a huge array of colours and make-up formulations. Plus a range of professional accessories, including sponges and brushes.

Crabtree & Evelyn

36 Milton Park

Abingdon

Oxfordshire OX14 4RT

tel 01235-862244

fax 01235-861222

http://www.crabtree-evelyn.com

Flower-, fruit- and herb-based toiletries, skincare products and fine fragrances. The range has recently been expanded and now includes a comprehensive aromatherapy collection.

Harrods

87–135 Brompton Road

Knightsbridge

London SW1 7XL

tel 020-7730 1234;

0845-6051234 (mail order)

A wide range of skincare and cosmetic lines, including Origins and Lancaster.

Dr Hauschka at Elysia

15 College Road

Bromsgrove

Worcestershire B60 2NF

tel/fax 01527-832863

Specialist skincare line based on herbal and floral waters that includes products designed to treat skin conditions.

Honesty Cosmetics

Lumford Mill

Unit 8

Buxton Road

Bakewell

Derbyshire DE45 1GS

tel 01629-814888

fax 01629-814111

Products from companies pursuing compassionate policies, including Beauty Without Cruelty and Deodorant Stone (the natural deodorant line).

Jo Malone

The Old Imperial Laundry

Warriner Gardens

London SW11 4XW

tel 020-7720 0202

fax 020-7720 0277

Specialist skincare line and own-label fragrances. Will also send gift-wrapped scents to friends or family.

Johnny Loves Rosie

32–38 Osborn Street

London E1 6TD

tel 020-7247 1496

fax 020-7247 3166

Comprehensive selection of the latest hair accessories, including decorative flower clips and headbands.

Kiehl's

tel 020-7379 7030 (UK mail order)

Hugely popular New York-based hair- and skincare range made with large quantities of natural ingredients. Some make-up colours also available.

Liz Earle by Mail

PO Box 50

Ryde

Isle of Wight

PO33 2YD

tel 01983-565222

fax 01983-812333

The celebrated health and beauty presenter's compact but effective range of cleansers, toners, skin polishers and moisturizers is available through mail order or on the QVC cable TV shopping channel.

Lush

29 High Street
Poole
Dorset BH15 1AB
tel 01202-668545
fax 01202-661832
Handmade soaps, lotions and bath products, plus some unusual fragrances and accessories. Gift boxes are also available.

Martha Hill

The Old Vicarage
Laxton
Corby
Northamptonshire NN17 3AT
tel 01780-450284
fax 01780-450398
Family-run herbal skincare company offering a wide range of face and body products.

Muji

187 Oxford Street
London W1R 1AJ
tel 020-7323 2208
No-fuss bath, body and haircare lines, plus handy packaging and some useful storage ideas.

The Natural Body Care Company

43 Cottonmill Lane
St Albans
Hertfordshire AL1 2BT
tel/fax 01727-839800
http://natural-bodycare.com
Toiletries and skincare products for women and men, babies and children.

Neal's Yard Remedies

Unit 1
St James House
St James Square
John Dalton Street
Manchester M2 6NY
tel/fax 0161-831 7875
Apothecary-style products for skin, body and hair, based on aromatherapy, essential oils and organic floral waters.

L'Occitane

237 Regent Street
London W1R 7AG
tel 020-7290 1421
fax 020-7290 1429
Beautiful essential oil-based range of skincare, bath and fragrance products, including traditional French soaps.

Opal London

65 Waterloo Road
London NW2 7TS
tel 020-8208 0708
fax 020-8450 3293
Beauty and bath accessories, including loofahs, scrubbing brushes, bath bags and shower caps.

Origins

Harrods
87–135 Brompton Road
Knightsbridge
London SW1 7XL
tel 020-7730 1234;
0845-6051234 (mail order)
Natural beauty products from America.

Penhaligon's by Request

PO Box 2888
London N4 1NH
tel 0800-716108
fax 020-8800 5789
Traditional fragrances and toiletries for both men and women. Gifts can also be delivered.

Les Petits Parfums

Freepost LON12152
London NW4 1YR
tel 020-8203 7521
fax 020-8905 8044
Fragrance miniatures to collect or sample without the expense of a whole new bottle. Brand names include Poppy Moreni, Oilily and Burberry.

Scent Direct Fragrances Worldwide

Freepost G13168
Haslemere
Surrey GU27 3BR
tel 01428-654575
A useful gift service that will wrap and deliver the fragrance of your choice.

Screenface

24 Powis Terrace
London W11 1JH
tel 020-7221 8289
fax 020-7792 9357
The make-up artists' favourite cosmetics haunt, with an extensive range of concealers and foundations as well as a great selection of make-up colours.

Les Senteurs

227 Ebury Street
London SW1W 8UT
tel 020-7730 2322
fax 020-7259 9145
Specialist perfumery for connoisseurs and those who want something a little out of the ordinary.

Shu Uemura

Unit 15–16 Thomas Neal's
29–41 Earlham Street
London WC2 9LD
tel 020-7379 6627
Comprehensive cosmetics collection that includes a wide range of colours and a huge choice of make-up brushes.

Space.NK.apothecary

PO Box 18025
London EC2A 3RJ
tel 0870-607706;
020-7636 2523 (for items not listed in the catalogue)
fax 020-7454 1153
Cutting edge boutique-style beauty and make-up lines, plus fragrance, skincare and haircare products for true beauty devotees. Ranges include Remède from New York's Bliss spa, Stila, Philosophy, Kiehl's and Antonia's Flowers fragrances.

Tisserand Aromatherapy Products

Unit 4
Newtown Road
Hove
Sussex BN3 7BA
tel 01273-325666
Specialists in aromatherapy and essential oils, with a wide selection of products that are suitable for both experts and beginners.

Tweezerman

Global Beauty Enterprises
4 Elephant Lane
London SE16 4JD
tel 020-7410 1667
fax 020-7410 1899
Professional beauty tools for skincare, manicures, eyebrow grooming and eyelash care.

Yves Rocher

664 Victoria Road
South Ruislip
Middlesex HA4 ONY
tel 020-8845 1222
fax 020-8845 1023
Long-established French toiletry and skincare range that includes a multitude of sweet-smelling goodies.

Helplines

Contact the following for expert advice.

Acne Support Group
tel 020-8561 6868
Medical advice for severe problem skins.

Aveda
tel 020-7410 1600
Skincare, colour and haircare hotline.

Bharti Vyas
tel 020-7486 7910
Expert holistic health and beauty advice.

British Association of
Electrolysists
tel 01895-239966/01708-226625
Information relating to electrolysis.

Carole Franck
tel 01823-421310
Salon details, plus advice on semi-
permanent make-up for brows and lips.

Clairol Advisory Service
tel 0800-181184
Haircare, styling and colouring advice.

La Formule
tel 01705-499133
Specialist skincare company that offers
advice for problem skins.

The International Federation
of Aromatherapy
tel 020-8742 2605
Advice on aromatherapy and the correct
use of essential oils.

Karin Herzog's Skincare
Advice Line
tel 0800-0562428
Skincare advice and recommendations.

Mavala Hotline
tel 01732-459412
Expert advice on nails and nailcare.

Shu Uemura
Unit 15–16
Thomas Neal's
29–41 Earlham Street
London WC2 9LD
tel 020-7379 6627

The Urban Retreat
4th Floor
Harvey Nichols
109–125 Knightsbridge
London SW1X 7R5
tel 020-7201 8610

Make-up courses

A make-up course is a good way to learn
new skills and get a feel for the industry.

Glauca Rossi School of Make-up
10 Sutherland Avenue
London W9 2HQ
tel 020-7289 7485
Four-, eight- and 12-week courses,
which include studio sessions with
photographers and models.

London College of Fashion
20 John Prince's Road
London W1M OBJ
tel 020-7514 7400 (full-time courses);
020-7514 7566 (part-time courses)
A range of courses, including a one-year
foundation course, two-year diploma
courses and a variety of evening classes.

London Esthetique
75–77 Margaret Street
London W1N 7HB
tel 020-7636 1893
Training days, plus short and long
courses with beauty professionals.

Makeovers

The companies listed below offer
make-up lessons or makeover sessions.
Telephone for details of appointments.

Carol Hayes
31 Great Marlborough Street
London W1V 1HA
tel 020-7287 1141

Cosmetics à la Carte
19b Motcomb Street
London SW1X 8LB
tel 020-7235 0596

The Face Place
33 Cadogan Street
London SW3 2PP
tel 020-7589 9062

The Green Room
tel 020-7376 0230 for details of your
nearest branch

Joy Goodman
21 Kingswood Avenue
London NW6 6LL
tel 020-8968 6887

Molton Brown
58 South Molton Street
London W1Y 1HH
tel 020-7499 6474

Screenface
24 Powis Terrace
London W11 1JH
tel 020-7221 8289

Facials

The following salons offer a range of
facials and other high-quality treatments.

Clarins Gold Salon
tel 020-7629 2979 for nearest branch
The premier league of Clarins salons.

Coopers
27 Maiden Lane
London WC2E 7JS
tel 020-7240 7170
Facials using Chinese skincare products.

Decleor Gold Salon
tel 020-7262 0403 for nearest branch
Essential oil-based treatments.

Elizabeth Arden's Red
Door Salon
29 Davies Street
London W1Y 3FN
tel 020-7629 4488
Cleansing and purifying facials and
rejuvenating treatments.

E'Spa Salon
tel 01252-741600 for nearest branch
A natural, holistic approach to skincare.

Guinot
tel 01344-873123 for nearest branch
Cathiodermie and other active skin
treatments that use hi-tech products.

L'Occitane
70 Kensington High Street
London W8 7PE
tel 020-7938 4135
Facials and makeovers using
L'Occitane's essential oil-based products.

Advice on the Internet

The following sites offer advice and information on the latest products, plus fun quizzes, tips and ideas for beauty devotees.

General

http://www.stylexperts.com

In-depth and light-hearted style tips covering fashion, food, homes and beauty. The site includes advice from model Niki Taylor, leading make-up artist Laura Mercier and top hairdresser Serge Norman. It also features supermodel and actress Iman, who has her own cosmetic and skincare range.

Skincare

Bioré

http://www.biore.com

Dynamic site that offers skincare quizzes, product-efficacy pages and answers to the most common beauty questions.

Blackmores

http://www.blackmores.com

Information on health and nutrition, including dietary tips and advice on vitamin supplements, free radicals and antioxidants. There's also an A–Z that covers everything from acne to pollution and stretchmarks.

The Body Shop

http://www.bodyshop.com

The beauty range with a conscience. The site explores human rights debates, offers question-and-answer pages about specific products, and has details of your nearest branch.

Cellex-C

http://www.cellex-c.com

Information on one of the first vitamin C skin-treatment ranges, with general advice, real-life before and after shots and up-to-date research.

Jurlique

http://www.jurlique.com

Details of this range of organic and bio-dynamic products.

Philosophy

http://www.philosophy.com

This dynamic American company reveals its philosophy – 'the beauty of every age' – and its range, which includes skincare, fragrances, make-up colours and bath products.

Make-up

Bobbi Brown Cosmetics

http://www.bobbibrowncosmetics.com

E-mail questions to make-up artist Bobbi herself, browse through her trade secrets and scour the archive of past tips. You can even order a catalogue from the site.

Cover Girl

http://www.covergirl.com

Your make-up questions answered. There are colour-matching pages for self-assessment, plus tips from top models and an e-mail page for your comments and questions.

Fashion Fair Cosmetics

http://www.fashioncosmetics.com

The biggest name in cosmetics for women with dark skins. The site has details of skincare, cosmetic and fragrance ranges, plus information on new products.

Hard Candy

http://www.hardcandy.com

Young and funky site offering an unbelievable range of colours. There's also a catalogue request service.

Urban Decay

http://www.urbandecay.com

Discover this anarchic selection of nail colours, eyeshadows and lipsticks, and order the products themselves. The site also features a biography of Sandy Lerner, the extraordinary woman behind the range.

Nails

Barielle

http://www.barielle.com

Information on nail and skincare products that have evolved from a treatment for horses' hooves. Plus order forms and stockist details.

Sally Hansen

http://www.sallyhansen.com

Submit questions to Hansen's regular expert Dr Scher on nail health and care. The magazine-style site also shows you how to achieve the perfect manicure at home as well as bringing you the latest nail colours and treatments. Plus free gifts and special offers.

Hair

Jo Hansford

http://www.johansford.com

The sought-after colour specialist offers advice on caring for coloured hair, plus helpful hints for aspiring hair colourists. Also details of how to become a house model and have your hair cut and coloured for free.

Joico

http://www.joico.com

International hair trends, plus a round-up of Joico's professional haircare products.

Vidal Sassoon

http://www.vidalsassoon.com

Hair and beauty experts offer advice, makeovers, plus the latest trends and ideas. You can also use the images featured to discover new styles that will work for you.

Cosmetic houses

Clinique

http://www.clinique.com

A great all-round site. There are answers to skincare queries, plus tips on camouflaging everything from broken capillaries to birthmarks. There's also a feedback page for e-mail questions, information on all the latest products and a bridal guide, complete with a quiz, tips and bridal traditions from around the world.

Lancôme

http://www.lancome.com

A busy site that includes chat from the Lancôme house models and the chance to create your own make-up looks on the virtual beauty pages. Worth visiting are the see, smell, touch and listen zones, which offer a variety of added extras, such as cocktail recipes.

Revlon

http://www.revlon.com

Virtual faces allow you to experiment with colours without going anywhere near a make-up counter. There are also giveaways, tools and tips. Plus you can download your very own Revlon vintage advertising image as a screensaver.

Perfume

Acqua Di Parma

http://www.acquadiparma.it

The famous Italian eau de cologne house introduces its upmarket bath and home accessories range.

Fragrance Counter

http://www.fragrancecounter.com

A user's guide to fragrance presented in an A–Z format. Answer the quiz questions and the on-screen advisers will identify a selection of fragrances that you might like to try.

Index

Picture credits

The author and publishers wish to thank these photographers, models and organizations for their kind permission to reproduce the following photographs in this book:

1 Greg Delves

2 Graham Shearer

  (Liisa Winkler for IMG)

4–11 Mitchell Sams

12 Pascal Chevallier

14–18 Mel Yates

20–21 Sarah Maingot

22 Mitchell Sams

25 Gillian Wong for Select

26–27 Alan Beukers

  (Marguerita Suppini for Boss)

28 Elliston Lutz

30–31 Rapid Eye

32–41 Sarah Maingot

43 Mel Yates

44–45 Rapid Eye

46 Sarah Maingot

(Yasmin Rossi)

48–49 Sarah Maingot

50 Sarah Maingot

  (Melanie Thierry for Select)

52–55 Graham Atkins Hughes

  (make-up by Jenny Jordan)

56–58 Mitchell Sams;

59 Mitchell Sams

  (Amber Valletta for Elite/Special Agent Management for Elizabeth Arden)

61–67 Mel Yates

68–69 Rapid Eye

71 Mitchell Sams

72–73 Graham Atkins Hughes

  (make-up by Jenny Jordan)

75 Ian Skelton

76–77 Rapid Eye

78–81 Graham Atkins Hughes

  (make-up by Jenny Jordan)

83 Nick Briggs

84–85 Graham Atkins Hughes

  (make-up by Jenny Jordan)

86–88 Alan Beukers

90 Mitchell Sams

93 Iain Crawford

  (Charlie Waterman for Models One)

94–95 Rapid Eye

96 Grey Zisser

98–99 Rapid Eye

100–109 Sarah Maingot

110–115 Graham Atkins Hughes

  (make-up by Jenny Jordan)

118 Mitchell Sams

121 Heribert Brehm

122–124 Sarah Maingot

125 Sarah Maingot

  (Lauren Gold for Select)

126–129 Rapid Eye;

130–135 Sarah Maingot;

136–139 Graham Atkins Hughes

  (make-up by Jenny Jordan)

140 Mitchell Sams

142 Grey Zisser

145 Mel Yates

152 Mitchell Sams

Author's acknowledgements

With thanks to:

Juliet Warkentin for getting me involved with the project – a very special thanks.

Suzanne Sykes for her inspirational input.

Susanna Cohen and Laurence Chevallier-Appert for their loyal assistance and hard work.

The photographers who worked so hard: Sarah Maingot, Mel Yates, Matt Anker and Graham Atkins Hughes.

The make-up artists, Jenny Jordan and Jo Karsberg, who not only contributed to the book but whose expertise has been so crucial over the years.

Andrew Roberts for the additional picture research.

Juliet Matthews and Rachel Pearce for the constant back-up.

Mark and Duff Westmoreland for all the moral support – extra special thanks.

Editorial Director: Jane O'Shea
Consultant Art Director: Helen Lewis
Project Editor: Pauline Savage
Text Editor: Kate Elms
Design Assistants: Coralie Bickford-Smith and Shoba Mucha
Production: Vincent Smith and Candida Jackson

First published in 1999 by Quadrille Publishing Ltd,
Alhambra House, 27–31 Charing Cross Road, London WC2H 0LS

This paperback edition first published in 2004

This book is published in association with European Magazines Ltd.

Cataloguing in Publication Data: a catalogue record for this book is available from the British Library.

ISBN 1 84400 076 1

Printed by Star Standard, Singapore

**Respiratory
Medicine**

CLINICAL CASES UNCOVERED

This book is dedicated to Belinda Brewer and her thirst for lifelong learning

Respiratory Medicine

CLINICAL CASES UNCOVERED

Emma H. Baker

PhD, FRCP

Reader in Clinical Pharmacology and Consultant Physician
St George's, University of London
London, UK

Dilys Lai

MD, MRCP

Consultant in Respiratory and General Medicine
Chelsea and Westminster Hospital
London, UK

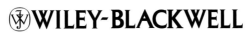

WILEY-BLACKWELL

A John Wiley & Sons, Ltd., Publication

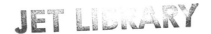

This edition first published 2008, © 2008 by E. H. Baker and D. Lai

Blackwell Publishing was acquired by John Wiley & Sons in February 2007. Blackwell's publishing program has been merged with Wiley's global Scientific, Technical and Medical business to form Wiley-Blackwell.

Registered office: John Wiley & Sons Ltd, The Atrium, Southern Gate, Chichester, West Sussex, PO19 8SQ, UK

Editorial offices: 9600 Garsington Road, Oxford, OX4 2DQ, UK
        The Atrium, Southern Gate, Chichester, West Sussex, PO19 8SQ, UK
        111 River Street, Hoboken, NJ 07030-5774, USA

For details of our global editorial offices, for customer services and for information about how to apply for permission to reuse the copyright material in this book please see our website at www.wiley.com/wiley-blackwell

Library of Congress Cataloguing-in-Publication Data

Baker, Emma.
Respiratory medicine : clinical cases uncovered / Emma Baker, Dilys Lai.
p. ; cm.
Includes index.
ISBN 978-1-4051-5895-4 (alk. paper)
1. Respiratory organs–Diseases–Case studies. 2. Respiratory organs–Diseases–Examinations, questions, etc. I. Lai, Dilys. II. Title.
[DNLM: 1. Respiratory Tract Diseases–Case Reports. 2. Respiratory Tract Diseases–Problems and Exercise. 3. Signs and Symptoms, Respiratory–Case Reports. 4. Signs and Symptoms, Respiratory–Problems and Exercises. WF 18.2 B167r 2008]
RC732.B34 2008
616.2–dc22
2007050635

ISBN: 978-1-4051-5895-4

A catalogue record for this book is available from the British Library

Set in 9/12pt Minion by SNP Best-set Typesetter Ltd., Hong Kong

Printed in Singapore by COS Printers Pte Ltd

1   2008